CONTENTS

Editor's Foreword: J A Horne

Chairman: Professor A H Crisp
Professor of Psychiatry
St George's Hospital Medical School
London

The use and abuse of hypnotics
M Lader   1

Why do old people complain of poor sleep?
K Morgan   11

Sleep disorders in childhood and adolescence
P Hill   20

Narcolepsy and the hypersomnias
J D Parkes   40

Sleep apnoea and snoring
J Stradling   46

Functions of sleep
J A Horne   61

List of delegates   74

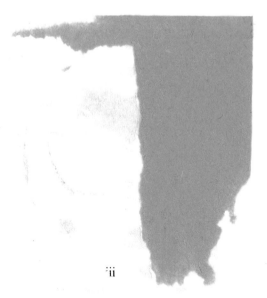

ii

EDITOR'S FOREWORD

For many physicians the term 'sleep disorder' is simply synonymous with insomnia, which is seen as a relatively minor ailment, and consequently the whole area tends to be relegated. Nevertheless, insomnia is a common complaint, causing anguish to many patients, and is not so amenable to drug therapy as is often believed. Although the reasons why we sleep are still somewhat of a mystery, many patients, especially insomniacs, worry about not getting their eight hours worth each night, and fear for their health as a consequence. This fear seems to be unfounded, and most do get adequate amounts of sleep. Early morning awakening and sleep disturbance are particularly prominent in the elderly. However, these symptoms reflect not so much an illness but part of the normal ageing process, not necessarily requiring treatment as such, but enlightenment. The same often applies to the parents of children who will not sleep, where simple behavioural approaches can have remarkably good outcomes.

There are, of course, more debilitating sleep disorders, particularly narcolepsy and those related to breathing, or rather cessation of breathing. These are more common than many physicians believe, where most sufferers go largely misdiagnosed or unnoticed.

The aim of this symposium, one of the first of its kind held in the UK, was to pursue some of these issues by getting together the leading specialists. Sleep disorders medicine has become a rapidly growing speciality in the USA and much of Europe, with numerous clinics, a standard nosology of over fifty sleep disorders, and its own professional regulatory organization. This is not to say that in the UK we are behind the times, but that we need to awaken to these developments.

J A HORNE
Director
Sleep Research Laboratory
Department of Human Sciences
Loughborough University

THE USE AND ABUSE OF HYPNOTICS

M Lader
Professor of Clinical Psychopharmacology
Institute of Psychiatry
University of London

Hypnotics are widely used drugs. About 17 million prescriptions were written for these compounds, mostly benzodiazepines, in Great Britain in 1985. In that year the prescriptions for hypnotics just outnumbered those for anxiolytics and sedatives which had dropped from about 24 million in 1975. Prescriptions for hypnotics have remained constant over the years. It must be presumed that the concern over long term usage and dependence which underlies the halving of tranquilliser prescriptions has not extended to the hypnotics. Is this perception of relative safety justified or is it another example of our complacency—of assuming that well-established drugs with wide usage could not possibly present a hazard? In this article I shall review the usage of hypnotic drugs and then deal with the possible problems which such usage entails.

INDICATIONS FOR HYPNOTICS

Sleep occupies a third of our lives and yet remains utterly mysterious. Studies in sleep laboratories have elucidated the physiology of sleep but not its purpose. The clinical importance of sleep reflects the frequency and severity of complaints of insomnia. Insomnia is taken to mean unsatisfactory or insufficient sleep, but subjectively, the patient complains of being awake when he should be asleep, and of feeling tired the next day.[1]

The classification of insomnia is complex,[2] but for the purposes of hypnotic use, the practitioner encounters three main types:[3]

1. Transient insomnia—'normal sleepers who experience an acute stress or stressful situation lasting several days (e.g., air travel to a new time zone or hospitalisation for elective surgery) that affects their sleep adversely.'
2. Short-term insomnia—'usually associated with a situational stress (e.g., acute personal loss) often related to work and family life or serious medical illness.'
3. Long-term insomnia—'available data suggest that insomnia in one third to one half of the patients in this category is related to underlying psychiatric conditions. A second group consists of persons whose insomnia is related to chronic drug-alcohol dependence or abuse.'

The strong consensus is that: 'Patients should receive the smallest effective dose of hypnotics for the shortest clinically necessary period of time': this recommendation applies especially to the elderly. Whether drugs should be used at all is more contentious. For transient insomnia, no consensus has emerged; for short-term insomnia, non-drug measures are recommended, at least at first; for chronic insomnia, careful enquiry and investigation are essential before drugs are prescribed. The last type of insomnia is the most complicated to treat,[4] and non-pharmacological techniques are being developed.[5]

TYPES OF HYPNOTICS

Although more complicated classifications have been suggested,[6] hypnotic drugs, primarily benzodiazepines, are generally divided into three groups.[7]

1. Short-acting, with mean elimination half-lives less than 6 hours. Examples include triazolam, midazolam and brotizolam.
2. Medium-acting, 6–12 hours, such as temazepam, lormetazepam and loprazolam.
3. Long-acting, over 12 hours with nitrazepam, flurazepam and flunitrazepam being in this category.

Further data are set out in table 1.

TABLE 1. Plasma elimination half-lives of hypnotic benzodiazepines and active metabolites in healthy subjects (from Jochemsen & Breimer, 1983)[8]

Compound	Elimination half-lives of parent drug (h) (mean + range or s.d.)	Active metabolite	Elimination half-life of metabolite (h)
Brotizolam	5.0 (3.1–6.1)	1-methylhydroxy-derivative	short
Flunitrazepam	15 (9–25)	7-amino-derivative	23
		N-desmethyl-derivative	31
Flurazepam	very short	N-desalkylflurazepam	87 (40–144)
		Hydroxyethyl-derivative	short
Lormetazepam	9.9 ± 2.4	—	—
Loprazolam	6.3 (4–8)	?	?
Midazolam	2.5 (1–3)	1-methylhydroxy-derivative	short
Nitrazepam	28 (20–34)	—	—
Temazepam	12 (8–21)	—	—
Triazolam	2.3 (1.4–3.3)	1-methylhydroxy-derivative	short

h = hours

As can be seen from Table 1, some compounds have significant metabolites with longer half-lives. Others in single dose are short acting because of a rapid

2

and marked redistribution phase, despite having long acting metabolites; diazepam is such a drug. A further important point is that the pharmaco-kinetics of many drugs are altered in the elderly. Usually there is a prolonged half-life and increased tissue sensitivity.[9]

EFFECTIVENESS OF HYPNOTICS

Many studies attest to the effects of hypnotics on sleep. Newer hypnotics have been extensively evaluated in sleep laboratories with respect to standard variables such as sleep latency, wake time after sleep onset and total wake time. In clinical studies evaluations have been with respect to subjective measures relating to estimates of time to fall asleep, 'quality of sleep' and feeling refreshed on awakening and later in the day. Reviews of various hypnotics have been published e.g. temazepam,[10] triazolam,[11] and loprazolam.[12]

In general, the efficacy of the hypnotics, at least in the short-term, is well-established. The type of efficacy accords quite well with the pharmacokinetic properties of each drug. For example, temazepam which is slowly absorbed has only marginal effects on sleep latency. Furthermore, the effects discerned in sleep laboratory studies are translated into clinically useful effects.

One point which does emerge from the numerous studies is the weakness of dose-response relationships. Each hypnotic has a minimally effective dose but often doubling the dose only increases side effects without materially improving efficacy.

Many benzodiazepine and other hypnotics seem to lose efficacy in laboratory studies after two weeks or so. Sleep latency shows more tolerance than does wake time. However, efficacy was largely maintained in the large-scale clinical studies, a puzzling paradox. Perhaps lying awake becomes less anxiety-provoking.

The efficacy of hypnotics is tempered by a range of unwanted effects which will not be reviewed.

RESIDUAL EFFECTS

Residual or 'hangover' effects comprise both subjective feelings of sedation and objective evidence of psychomotor and cognitive impairment occurring during the day after the ingestion of an hypnotic drug the previous night.[13] A range of measures is available to assess these effects.[14] Sometimes subjects may feel normal and yet show objective impairment.

Again, as with efficacy, residual effects are fairly well-predicted from the pharmacokinetics of each drug, providing both the redistribution and elimination phases are considered. Because of altered pharmacokinetics, residual effects are usually more marked in the elderly and may result in falls, immobility, restlessness and confusion.[15]

Dosage is an important consideration. Any hypnotic in high enough dosage will produce residual effects, whatever its half-life; even the long-acting agents may be devoid of detectable residual effects at low dosage.

3

Residual effects are easier to detect in normal subjects than in insomniac patients. Perhaps the mild sedation present the next morning is welcomed by some patients as a relief from their constant anxiety. Tolerance is also an important factor.

Residual effects may also take the form of 'crises' such as a car crash or outbursts of irritability. These have been well-described by Oswald's group.[16]

REBOUND INSOMNIA

This has been defined by one group as a 'statistically significant increase or an increase of 40% or greater in the mean group value for total wake time for a single withdrawal night or the entire withdrawal condition as compared to baseline'.[17] Other investigators measure it in terms of statistical significance for sleep latency or wake time. Absolute rebound is an increase in these variables above pretreatment levels. However, other changes may be clinically relevant, such as those from final drug administration to early withdrawal and from early withdrawal to late withdrawal. A 'relative' rebound insomnia may occur between these nights of the study without reverting to baseline levels.

Both sleep laboratory studies and clinical evaluations can assess the presence of rebound. The former are precise but are carried out in artificial conditions; the latter are real-life assessments but rely on subjective recordings of dubious validity.

A plethora of studies has established that rebound insomnia is a real phenomenon. What is more controversial is the relationship between the incidence and severity of rebound insomnia and the effective duration of action of the hypnotic. Claims that rebound insomnia is commoner and more severe after discontinuing short—or intermediate—acting drugs than long-acting drugs, have not been universally accepted.[18] However, a recent review of the literature[19] concluded 'that rebound insomnia is most clearly established after the withdrawal of short-acting benzodiazepines, and is also most severe, but also the shortest lived; it is also discernible after the withdrawal of intermediate-acting benzodiazepine hypnotics, but may be delayed for 2 or more nights; it may be less severe but more prolonged or it may occur on a sporadic basis following the withdrawal of the very long-acting compounds.' In general, the peak withdrawal effect is related to the elimination half-life of the compound.

Equally important are dosage considerations. Clear dose-effect relationships can be discerned, e.g. 0.5 mg of triazolam is associated with rebound, whereas no rebound was seen after 0.25 mg triazolam.[20] The key question is whether rebound insomnia occurs to a clinically significant extent at usual dosages. No data address this issue directly but studies have suggested that rebound insomnia is a factor in the routine use of hypnotics in the longer term.[21] As duration of usage does not seem to be an important factor, it seems that rebound insomnia may occur with almost all hypnotics unless the dosage is kept minimal. Older patients may be particularly at risk.

4

OTHER REBOUND PHENOMENA

Two other clinical syndromes have been reported and attributed to a rebound mechanism. Early morning insomnia consists of a worsening of sleep that occurs during the final hours of the night during actual drug administration.[22] It is seen with short-acting hypnotics such as triazolam. It was proposed that this syndrome represented rebound during each night of administration due to the clearance of the drug from its receptors by early morning. A similar phenomenon is seen with alcohol, which is metabolised at a rapid but constant rate (zero-order kinetics) and is associated with broken sleep during the latter part of the night.

A related syndrome is that of daytime anxiety. Some studies[23] have reported increases in ratings of anxiety during the day during the administration of short- and even intermediate-acting benzodiazepines. Longer-acting compounds do not seem to be associated with this effect.

DEPENDENCE

A coruscatingly detailed review,[24] (1987) of benzodiazepine dependence concluded that the research evidence supports the claim that:

(a) physiological dependence to benzodiazepines does occur.
(b) the withdrawal signs seem more severe after high dose than low dose usage.
(c) dependence can develop to therapeutic doses if the drugs are given long-term.
(d) withdrawal signs develop more rapidly and may be more severe following chronic administration of shorter-acting rather than longer-acting benzodiazepines.
(e) dependence does not occur in all chronic users.
(f) concomitant or prior use of drugs such as barbiturates or ethanol may increase the likelihood of development of dependence on the benzodiazepines.

Withdrawal symptoms from anxiolytic benzodiazepines have been described in detail (e.g.)[25] Less attention has been paid to the hypnotic benzodiazepines. These compounds are identical pharmacologically to the anxiolytic drugs, their usage as sleeping tablets reflecting commercial rather than scientific considerations. Consequently, one would expect all these compounds to be capable of inducing dependence. The only difference might be that the dosing interval of 24 hours with a hypnotic might militate against the development of dependence.

The acceptance of rebound insomnia as a complication of hypnotic benzodiazepine use should lead us to reassess the dangers of a full-blown withdrawal syndrome on continued use. The distinction between the two is arbitrary, withdrawal usually being regarded as containing symptoms other than insomnia. Thus, withdrawal from a hypnotic will comprise fearfulness, restlessness, excess REM sleep and bizarre dreams, the last even breaking into wakefulness as paranoid ideas, fears and delusions or as hallucinations and clouding of consciousness.[26] Clinical accounts of withdrawal syndromes after discontinuing benzodiazepines contain numerous instances of such features following discontinuation of hypnotics after long-term use.

USAGE OF HYPNOTICS

Against this background we can now seek to establish usage rates of hypnotics in the UK and attempt to conclude whether such usage is justified or alarming. Data are available from several sources but all are subject to various limitations.[24]

Surveys of prescriptions show that sedatives and hypnotics have remained fairly steady at about 15% of the total for all drugs for the past 40 years. However, this represents an absolute increase, as prescriptions in general have increased in number over the years. Usage in the UK is now about average in the Western world with about 46 million dosage units being prescribed for an adult population of 45 million. In 1984, the most popular hypnotic by far was nitrazepam, with 2.5 times the market share of temazepam. Flurazepam and triazolam were next. However, the 'Limited List' has since been brought in from which flurazepam is absent. The most notable change in patterns of prescribing concerns the replacement of the barbiturates by the benzodiazepines.

As mentioned earlier, prescriptions for anxiolytic, but not hypnotic, benzodiazepines have fallen over the past decade.

A survey of general practice patients found that about a quarter of those taking hypnotics regularly had started taking them during a hospital stay. Another survey suggested that such usage had decreased between the 1970's and the 1980's.

Community surveys have indicated that insomnia is the most frequently cited reason for starting to take a benzodiazepine. The proportion of people reporting insomnia and taking hypnotics increased with age; conversely, the proportion reporting 'nerves' etc. decreased with age. Long-term use of drugs increased with age; of all respondents aged 55 or over, 14% were taking psychotropic drugs on a long-term basis, compared with 3% of respondents aged between 18 and 34.

A recent survey involved data from 1020 randomly selected subjects aged 65 and over.[27] Of these 16% reported using an hypnotic drug, usually a benzodiazepine. Three-quarters of these had taken an hypnotic for more than one year, a quarter for more than 10 years. In other words, 12% of the elderly are chronic benzodiazepine users. The most frequently used drug was nitrazepam, although, its popularity seemed to be declining in favour of intermediate- and short-acting compounds.

In 1972 Clift[28] prospectively studied patients in a Manchester general practice, who presented with insomnia of recent origin. A year following the initial prescriptions, 32% were still receiving repeat prescriptions for the regular use of non-barbiturate hypnotics, mainly nitrazepam. After a further three years this prevalence had halved. Some other patients were intermittent users, relying on hypnotics at times of 'personal disturbance'. Admonitions to use hypnotics as sparingly as possible were quite effective, only 8% of users of this regimen were still coming for prescriptions at the end of a year.

Attempts have been made to relate such high and chronic usage to the severity and chronicity of insomnia.[29] Insomnia was found to afflict about a third of the population each year, particularly elderly women with psychic distress and somatic anxiety. Many did not receive medication. Most chronic insomniacs were either anxious or depressed, and the data from this and similar studies could be used to support the viewpoint that insomnia is a symptom which should not be treated separately but rather as part of psychiatric disorder.

ABUSE OF HYPNOTICS

This refers to the non-medical, recreational use of these drugs. The benzodiazepines have mild reinforcing effects which appear to be more pronounced in subjects who are known recreational users of other drugs. Benzodiazepines are used by various populations of abusers such as alcoholics and heroin addicts, typically to eke out their supply of their drug of first preference. Abuse of benzodiazepines alone is not common.

CONCLUSION

Hypnotics are widely-used medications although their only indication, insomnia, is an ill-defined complaint. Various types of insomnia exist, as do a variety of causes. Most short-term insomnia is associated with stress and can be alleviated by the short-term use of an hypnotic. Most long-term insomnia is associated with psychiatric disorders, drug- or alcohol-related problems. Careful investigation and evaluation are necessary before resorting to hypnotic medication in these patients.

REFERENCES

1 Dement W, Seidel W, Carskadon M. Issues in the diagnosis and treatment of insomnia. In: Hindmarch I, Ott H, Roth T, eds. *Psychopharmacology Supplement I*. Berlin Heidelberg: Springer-Verlag, 1984:11–43.
2 Cleghorn J M, Kaplan R D, Bellissimo A, Szatmari P. Insomnia: I. Classification, assessment and pharmaceutical treatment. *Can J Psychiatry* 1983;**28**:339–46.
3 Consensus Conference. Drugs and insomnia. The use of medications to promote sleep. *JAMA* 1984;**251**:2410–4.
4 Cleghorn J M, Bellissimo A, Kaplan R D, Szatmari P. Insomnia: II. Assessment and treatment of chronic insomnia. *Can J Psychiatry* 1983;**28**:347–53.
5 Killen J, Coates T J. The complaint of insomnia: what is it and how do we treat it? In: Franks C M, eds. *New Developments in behavior therapy: from research to clinical application*. New York: Haworth Press, 1984:377–408.
6 Nicholson A. Hypnotics. Their place in therapeutics. *Drugs* 1986;**31**:164–76.
7 Greenblatt D J, Divoll M, Abernethy D R, Shader R I. Benzodiazepine hypnotics: kinetic and therapeutic options. *Sleep* 1982;**5**:S18–27.
8 Breimer D D, Jochemsen R. Clinical pharmacokinetics of hypnotic benzodiazepines: a summary. *Br J Clin Pharmacol* 1983;**16**:277S–8S.

9 Hicks R, Dysken M W, Davis J M, Lesser J, Ripeckyj A, Lazarus L. The pharmacokinetics of psychotropic medication in the elderly: a review. *J Clin Psychiatry* 1981;**42**:374–85.

10 Heel R C, Brogden R N, Speight T M, Avery G S. Temazepam: A review of its pharmacological properties and therapeutic efficacy as an hypnotic. *Drugs* 1981;**21**:321–40.

11 Pakes G E, Brogden R N, Heel R C, Speight T M, Avery G S. Triazolam: a review of its pharmacological properties and therapeutic efficacy in patients with insomnia. *Drugs* 1981;**22**:81–110.

12 Clark B G, Jue S G, Dawson G W, Ward A. Loprazolam. A preliminary review of its pharmacodynamic and pharmacokinetic properties and therapeutic efficacy in insomnia. *Drugs* 1986;**31**:500–16.

13 Johnson L C, Chernik D A. Sedative-hypnotics and human performance. *Psychopharmacol* 1982;**76**:101–13.

14 Bond A, Lader M. After effects of sleeping drugs. In: Wheatley D, ed. *Psychopharmacology of Sleep*. New York: Raven Press, 1981:177–93.

15 Fancourt G, Castleden M. The use of benzodiazepines with particular reference to the elderly. *Br J Hosp Med* 1986;**35**(5):321–6.

16 Morgan K, Adam K, Oswald I. Effect of loprazolam and of triazolam on psychological functions. *Psychopharmacol* 1984;**82**:386–8.

17 Kales A, Soldatos C R, Bixler E O, Kales J D. Rebound insomnia and rebound anxiety: a review. *Pharmacology* 1983;**26**:121–37.

18 Kales A, Scharf M B, Kales J D, Soldatos C R. Rebound insomnia; a potential hazard following withdrawal of certain benzodiazepines. *JAMA* 1979;**241**(No. 16):1692–5.

19 Lader M, Lawson C. Sleep studies and rebound insomnia: methodological problems, laboratory findings, and clinical implications. *Clin Neuropharmacol* 1987;**10**:291–312.

20 Roehrs T A, Zorick F J, Wittig R M, Roth T. Dose determinants of rebound insomnia. *Br J Clin Pharmacol* 1986; **22**:143–7.

21 Oswald I, French D, Adam K, Gilham J. Benzodiazepine hypnotics remain effective for 24 weeks. *Br Med J* 1982;**284**:860–3.

22 Kales A, Soldatos C R, Bixler E O, Kales J D. Early morning insomnia with rapidly eliminated benzodiazepines. *Science* 1983;**220**:95–7.

23 Morgan K, Oswald I. Anxiety caused by a short-life hypnotic. *Br Med J* 1982;**284**: 942.

24 Woods J H, Katz J L, Winger G. Abuse liability of benzodiazepines. *Pharmacol Rev* 1987;**39**:251–419.

25 Petursson H, Lader M. *Dependence on tranquillizers*. Oxford: Oxford University Press, 1984.

26 Oswald I. Benzodiazepines and sleep. In: Trimble M R, ed. *Benzodiazepines Divided*. John Wiley & Sons, 1983:261–76.

27 Morgan K, Dallosso H, Ebrahim S, Arie T, Fentem P H. Prevalence, frequency and duration of hypnotic drug use among the elderly living at home. *Br Med J* 1988; **296**:601–2.

28 Clift A D. Factors leading to dependence on hypnotic drugs. *Br Med J* 19721;**3**: 614–7.

29 Mellinger G D, Balter M B, Uhlenhuth F H. Insomnia and its treatment. Prevalence and correlates. *Arch Gen Psychiatry* 1985;**42**:225–32.

DISCUSSION

Audience   Could I ask Professor Lader to comment on the present and future status of non benzodiazepine hypnotics?

Professor Lader   Many of the drugs in development, although chemically not benzodiazepines, act in a similar way. Therefore one has to consider whether they have the same profile of advantages and disadvantages as the benzodiazepines. Amongst the anxiolytics whole groups of compounds are being developed which act on the 5HT system which have anxiolytic properties, are less sedative and do not appear to have the same propensity for dependence. I know of no similar compounds in the offing in the field of hypnotics, the reason is probably that sedation is what is required of a hypnotic. They are unique in the sense that the wanted effect, sedation, and the unwanted effect, sedation, are only separated by 8 hours in time. More refined hypnotics, will be variations on a theme, compounds with perhaps a slightly different combination of properties.

We now have benzodiazepine antagonists. Perhaps we will reach the situation predicted in 'Brave New World', where people take sleeping tablets and then in the morning they take something else to wipe out the effect of the sleeping tablet; that is now technically feasible.

Audience   Have you noticed any beneficial effect of short acting versus intermediate acting benzodiazepines in terms of effects on memory?

Professor Lader   Benzodiazepines seem to vary in their propensity to affect memory. They all do the same sort of thing; in simple terms, they prevent short term memory going into long term memory, the traces are not stored. In certain circumstances the amnesic effect of benzodiazepines are a great boon; when performing an unpleasant investigation administering a benzodiazepine (as long as it does not interfere with the test) may be merciful. Some of these benzodiazepines have disproportionate effects on memory compared to others, for instance lorazepam produces effects on memory unlike closely related compounds like oxazepam.[1] Therefore there are certain compounds which are particularly devastating in terms of impairment of memory; so far lorazepam, and probably alprazolam have been identified. This does not seem to be related to half life. Perhaps this is to do with the receptor affinities of these drugs. Some compounds have a high affinity to benzodiazepine receptors, reflected in the fact that a low dose is required and also in certain properties which they exhibit, which are not seen to the same extent in other compounds used in similar doses. The effects on memory of the benzodiazepines do not show tolerance as quickly as effects on sedation, or effects on psychomotor ability.[2] Somebody who has been on a benzodiazepine for five years will still be suffering from memory impairment.

Dr Parkes   Can I just ask Professor Lader what drug to take, at what dose, and at what time, before going to the west coast of America and coming back?

9

Professor Lader If you insist on these adventurous trips, I would suggest that you take an intermediate acting agent such as lormetazepam in the smallest possible dose.

Dr Stradling Professor Lader, do you think sedation and sleep provocation cannot be separated? We hear about sleep provoking peptides and all that kind of thing. Do you really not think that sleep is different from sedation and that sedation merely makes you feel like going to sleep? Surely the sleep making mechanism is clearly different from sedation?

Professor Lader There have been attempts to look at compounds like peptides, which may have a specific effect on sleep, but the benzodiazepines are non specific cerebral depressants. Therefore if you are inducing sleep in an artificial way, which is a form of sedation, those two things cannot be separated. That does not mean that there may not be other ways of affecting sleep other than swamping the GABA mechanisms. I look forward to seeing these alternatives being developed but they are not going to be available in the foreseeable future.

REFERENCES

1 Curran H V, Schiwy W, Lader M. Differential amnesic properties of benzo-diazepines: a dose-response comparison of two drugs with similar elimination half-lives. *Psychopharmacology* 1987;**92**:358–64.
2 Lucki I, Rickels K, Geller A M. Chronic use of benzodiazepines and psychomotor and cognitive test performance. *Psychopharmacology* 1986;**88**:426–33.

WHY DO OLD PEOPLE COMPLAIN OF POOR SLEEP?

Kevin Morgan
Lecturer in Gerontology
Department of Health Care of the Elderly
University of Nottingham Medical School
Nottingham NG7 2UH

As a feature of the ageing process, deteriorating sleep quality has long attracted both clinical and literary attention. Writing in *The Lancet* in 1836, for example, Dr George Sigmond observed that 'The duration of sleep should be, in manhood, about the fourth or the sixth of the 24 hours; children, the younger they are the more sleep they require; in advanced age there is more watchfuless' (i.e. wakefulness).[1] Later that same century Herman Melville, in his novel *Moby Dick*, somewhat drily explained that 'Old age is always wakeful; as if, the longer linked with life, the less man has to do with aught that looks like death'.[2] While the novelist provides us with a little more food for thought, it is evident that both writer and clinician appreciated a connection between age and sleep. More recently this connection has been quantified in numerous population surveys conducted in a variety of geographical and cultural settings. Thus, from Kiev to Kuwait,[3] or from Florida[4] to Finland,[3] or from Glasgow[5] to rural Greece[3] dissatisfaction with sleep tends to increase with age.

Of course, reporting dissatisfaction with sleep during a community survey is not quite the same thing as complaining of sleeplessness. Nevertheless, this dissatisfaction frequently does translate into a complaint of insomnia. It is not particularly surprising therefore that the prescribing of hypnotics is also age-related and that, for at least the past thirty years, elderly people have remained the most likely target group for these drugs.[6] Recent estimates, for example, suggest that in Britain, up 1 million elderly people consume a hypnotic each night.[7] In addition to this increased prevalence, *patterns* of sleeping drug consumption also show an age-related change, with regular and protracted use becoming more common in old age. Unfortunately, most of the disadvantages associated with hypnotic drugs in the elderly are directly related to this style of consumption. Thus, confusional states,[8] impaired psychomotor performance,[9] increased daytime anxiety,[10] rebound insomnia,[11] and dependence[12] are all more likely if hypnotics are taken regularly over long periods of time.

Increasingly, however, the widespread use of benzodiazepine hypnotics and tranquillisers among vulnerable groups is becoming both socially and clinically unacceptable.[13] This growing concern emphasises the need for a broader and more flexible response to complaints of poor sleep in later life—a response which includes assessment, education, counselling, and the

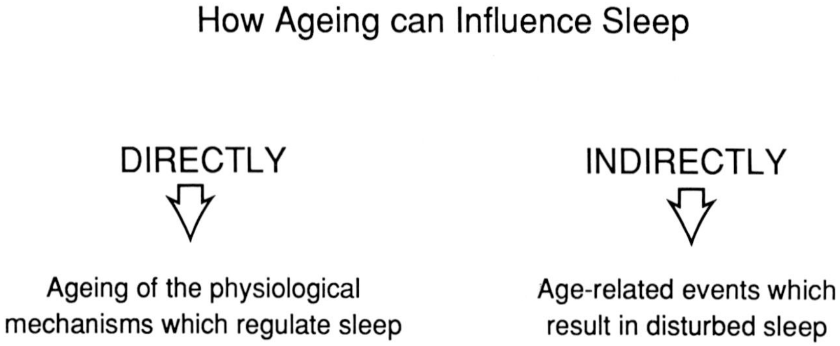

How Ageing can Influence Sleep

DIRECTLY	INDIRECTLY
⇩	⇩
Ageing of the physiological mechanisms which regulate sleep	Age-related events which result in disturbed sleep

FIGURE 1.

use, in particular, of psychological services. To be effective and appropriately targetted, a broader clinical response requires a clear understanding of the physical, social, and psychological factors which can mediate complaints of poor sleep in old age. Valuable contributions to such an understanding can, I believe, be gained by addressing the simple question which provides the title for this presentation: why do old people complain of poor sleep?

THE EFFECTS OF AGEING ON SLEEP

Conceptually, the process of ageing can influence sleep quality either directly or indirectly, as shown in Figure 1. Direct influences are those which are due, or are assumed to be due to the ageing of the nervous system and the physiological mechanisms which regulate sleep and waking (for example, the progressive decline in slow wave sleep throughout early and late adulthood). Indirect influences, on the other hand, can result either from age-related biological events (e.g. nocturia), or from age-related personal or social events (e.g. bereavement, poverty). While conceptually tidy, the categories shown in Figure 1 are not entirely distinct and, to some extent, overlap. It should also be remembered that, at any age, disruptive influences upon sleep are potentially additive, and events from one category can, and in old age frequently do, combine with events from another.

THE DIRECT INFLUENCE OF AGE

Since the discovery of REM periods in 1953,[14] and the subsequent upsurge of interest in all-night EEG recordings, numerous studies have reported that human sleep shows consistent age-related changes in continuity, duration, and depth. In so far as they occur in ostensibly healthy individuals and are not associated with known disease processes, these changes can be considered normal. Nevertheless, each of these changes has implications for subjective sleep quality.

Continuity

Brief periods of wakefulness during sleep are normal at any age. Often the individual is unaware of these arousals, and has no trouble in returning to sleep. With advancing age, however, these periods of wakefulness tend to become both more frequent[15] and longer[16], and can seriously degrade the perceived continuity of sleep.

Duration

Perhaps one of the most detailed analyses of ontogenetic changes in total daily sleep is that reported[17] (and since revised[18]) by Roffwarg and colleagues in 1966. In healthy adult volunteers average total daily sleep gradually falls from approximately 7.75 hours per day among those aged 19–30, to 6 hours or less among those aged 50–90. Even when daytime naps are taken into consideration, many healthy, well-adjusted individuals clearly sleep less as they grow older.[18]

Depth

With advancing age depth of sleep appears to be affected both quantitatively and qualitatively. Age-related changes in the architecture of sleep result in a diminution of deeper slow wave sleep (Stage 3 and 4), and a reciprocal increase in light sleep (Stage 2) and drowsiness (Stage 1).[14] Thus, older sleep is structurally—or quantitatively—lighter. In addition, studies of auditory awakening thresholds (or AATs—the minimum amount of noise required to arouse a sleeping person) show age-related qualitative changes in the depth of individual sleep stages. A study reported by Zepelin and colleagues[19], for example, shows that during stages 2, 4, and REM sleep, older people are more easily awakened by noise (i.e. have lower AATs) than are younger people (this despite audiometric assessments showing the older volunteers to have less sensitive hearing).

THE INDIRECT INFLUENCE OF AGE

Old age can also be accompanied by events which, while not directly related to the physiological mechanisms which regulate sleep, may nevertheless severely degrade sleep quality. These *indirect* influences may be sub-divided into the biological (or internal) and the social (or external), as shown in Figure 2. Both sub-categories include a diverse collection of factors which can impinge upon sleep in later life, some of which are presented in Table 1. Indirect factors may act singly, or in combination with others. Furthermore, whether internal or external, organic or personal, many of these factors will be superimposed upon existing age-related reductions in the continuity, duration, and depth of sleep. Clearly, then, Figure 2 emphasises not only the variety but also the complexity of events which can underlie disturbed sleep in later life.

How Ageing can Influence Sleep

DIRECTLY
$\Downarrow$

Ageing of the physiological
mechanisms which regulate sleep

INDIRECTLY
$\Downarrow$

Age-related events which
result in disturbed sleep

Biological events   Social events

FIGURE 2.

TABLE 1. Age-related factors which can influence quality of sleep indirectly

Biological (internal) Factors	Social (external) Factors
Changes in bladder function	Bereavement
Sleep disordered breathing	Living alone
Limb-movements during sleep	Financial hardship
Pain and physical discomfort	Institutionalisation
Iatrogenic causes	
Mental health:	
Depression	
Dementia	

OTHER FACTORS INFLUENCING SUBJECTIVE INSOMNIA IN OLD AGE

It is a not infrequent assumption that complaints which are prevalent *in* old age are somehow due *to* old age. Thus, high levels of subjective insomnia among elderly people are often exclusively attributed to the processes of ageing outlined in Figures 1 and 2, and briefly discussed above. This impression is, I think, reinforced by the data describing the epidemiology of insomnia which, almost without exception, describe prevalence rather than incidence. There are, however, both logical and practical limitations to the assumption that insomnia in old age is usually due to old age. Poor sleep is not entirely unknown in younger age-groups, and it is reasonable to suppose that many of these younger insomniacs grow old with their complaint. If this is the

14

case then it is also likely that some of the psychological characteristics which appear to discriminate between younger good and poor sleepers might also discriminate between elderly good and poor sleepers. This issue is not without clinical relevance.

ANXIETY AND NEUROTICISM AS RISK FACTORS FOR INSOMNIA

Studies in which the personality profiles of good and poor sleepers have been compared consistently show elevated levels of neuroticism and anxiety among subjective insomniacs.[20,21] The possibility exists, therefore, that stable anxiety-related personality characteristics act as risk factors for insomnia, and may interact with and (in some cases) exacerbate the impact of normal and pathological ageing. Thus, even where some evident age-related event may be perceived as the cause of disturbed sleep, constitutional levels of anxiety and neuroticism may contribute to the *complaint* of insomnia. Some elderly subjective insomniacs may, therefore, benefit from therapeutic interventions which focus on anxiety management. Unfortunately, much of the evidence linking personality and subjective sleep quality has been derived either from relatively young volunteers, or from small and highly selected elderly groups. As a result the role (if any) of personality in mediating persistent complaints of poor sleep within the general elderly population remains unclear, and the value of anxiety management in such cases remains speculative.

Recently, however, some of these issues have been clarified by data from the Nottingham Longitudinal Study of Activity and Ageing—a project set up in 1984 specifically to investigate the role of physical activity and lifestyle in promoting and maintaining wellbeing in old age. In this context, sleep quality was identified as an important index of both physical and psychological wellbeing. Briefly, data were collected as follows: of 1299 individuals randomly sampled from the community and invited to participate in the study, 1042 (80%) agreed, and were interviewed in their own homes in 1985.[22] Within this stratified random sample (507 aged 65–74; 535 aged 75 +), 105 (21%) of the younger age group, and 130 (25%) of the older age group reported problem sleep 'often or all the time'. While the study has provided considerable information on various aspects of sleep and hypnotic drug use,[7,23] only two issues need concern us here: first, when do elderly poor sleepers actually *become* poor sleepers? and second, is the complaint of poor sleep in old age related to personality?

WHEN DO ELDERLY POOR SLEEPERS BECOME POOR SLEEPERS?

Follow-up interviews of subjective insomniacs in the younger age-group (i.e. those aged between 65 and 74) were conducted some two years after the original data collection. While including many of the original questions

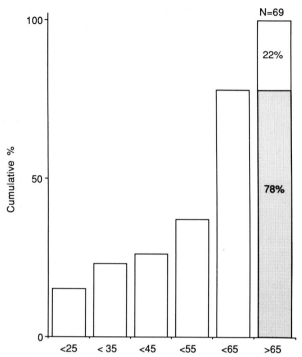

FIGURE 3. Estimated age of onset of persistent subjective insomnia in 69 poor sleepers aged 65–74

concerning sleep, the structured follow-up interviews also included psychometric assessments of personality (using the Eysenck Personality Questionnaire—EPQ) and anxiety (using the Speilberger State/Trait Anxiety Inventory—STAI).[24] Of the original 105 insomniac respondents 82 were re-interviewed and, of these, 69 (85%) continued to complain of poor sleep. We therefore nominated this sub-group 'persistent subjective insomniacs'.

Information provided at the follow-up interviews allowed us to estimate the age of each of these individuals at the onset of their perceived sleep disturbance. The cumulative distribution of these ages is shown in Figure 3. Interestingly, a substantial proportion of these insomniacs had become dissatisfied with their sleep before the onset of middle age. Indeed, if we adopt the (quite arbitrary) convention of dividing the elderly from the non-elderly at age 65, then it can be seen that 78% of these respondents had become insomniac before they had become elderly. Clearly, then, events and processes associated with old age cannot fully explain the prevalence of subjective insomnia in this representative sample of 'young' elderly persistent insomniacs.

IS POOR SLEEP RELATED TO PERSONALITY IN OLD AGE?

Persistent subjective insomniacs were then age and sex matched with a randomly selected group of 'stable good sleepers' who, at both the original and follow-up interviews, reported that they never or seldom had problems sleeping. Of the many variables considered, discriminant function analysis showed that only three factors significantly discriminated between the two groups, viz. neuroticism (from the EPQ), tea consumption, and the total number of drugs prescribed (the latter providing an index of general health status). Thus, the subjective insomniacs showed elevated levels of neuroticism, higher levels of tea consumption, and appeared to be less physically healthy, than their non-insomniac contemporaries.[24] (It should be pointed out that, in bivariate comparisons the poor sleepers also showed significantly elevated levels of both state and trait anxiety. In the multivariate analysis, however, these factors did not contribute significantly to the discriminant function once neuroticism was controlled.)

Interestingly, while the contribution of health status and tea drinking (the latter having both stimulant and diuretic effects) to the complaint of poor sleep is predicted from the schema shown in Figure 2, the contribution of anxiety-related personality factors is not. Nor does it appear to be the case that neuroticism results from, rather than contributes to poor sleep. Rather, both the neuroticism scale from the EPQ, and the trait anxiety scale from the STAI are assumed to reflect stable personality characteristics, rather than transient, reactive mood changes.

SOME CONCLUSIONS

Perhaps for too long the simple expedient of prescribing hypnotic drugs has encouraged a clinically simplistic conceptualisation of sleep problems in old age. It is clear, however, that with advancing age subjective insomnia becomes increasingly multifactorial in origin, with ill health, changing personal circumstances, and ontogenetic changes in the structure of sleep all playing a part. In addition, many elderly insomniacs do not develop their sleep problem in later life but rather 'graduate' into old age with a pre-existing history of poor quality sleep—thus admitting the possibility of clinically distinct sub-types of subjective insomnia in old age (for example 'graduate' insomniacs as distinct from 'old age onset' insomniacs). This, together with the further possibility that aspects of personality may act as risk factors for complaints of poor sleep at any age, requires further research attention. Ideally, such research should be aimed, not at needlessly quantifying the vicissitudes of later life, but at realistically matching causes of insomnia with effective clinical responses.

REFERENCES

1 Sigmond G G. Lectures on materia medica and therapeutics. *Lancet* 1836;**37(1)**: 214–20.
2 Melville H. *Moby Dick*. London, 1851:29.

3 Heikkinen E, Waters W E, Brzezinski Z J, eds. *The elderly in eleven countries: a sociomedical survey*. WHO Regional Office for Europe; Copenhagen; 1983.

4 Karacan I, Thornby J I, Anch M, *et al*. The prevalence of sleep disturbance in a primarily urban Florida county. *Social Science and Medicine* 1976;**10**:239–44.

5 McGhie A, Russell S M. The subjective assessment of normal sleep patterns. *Journal of Mental Science* 1962;**108**:642–54.

6 Morgan K. Sedative-hypnotic drug use and ageing. *Archives of Gerontology and Geriatrics* 1983;**2**:181–99.

7 Morgan K, Dallosso H, Ebrahim S, Arie T, Fentem P H. Prevalence, frequency, and duration of hypnotic drug use among the elderly living at home. *British Medical Journal* 1988;**296**:601–2.

8 Evans J G, Jarvis E H. Nitrazepam and the elderly. *British Medical Journal* 1972;**4**:487.

9 Morgan K. Effects of repeated dose nitrazepam and lormetazepam on psycho-motor performance in the elderly. *Psychopharmacology* 1985;**86**:209–11.

10 Morgan K, Oswald I. Anxiety caused by a short life hypnotic. *British Medical Journal* 1982;**284**:942.

11 Oswald I, Adam K, Borrow S, Idzikowski C. The effects of two hypnotics on sleep, subjective feelings and skilled performance. In: Passouant P, Oswald I, eds. *Pharmacology of the states of alertness*. Oxford: Pergamon Press, 1979:51–63.

12 Higgit A C, Lader M H, Fonagy P. Clinical management of benzodiazepine dependence. *British Medical Journal* 1985;**291**:688–90.

13 See, for example, Committee on Safety of Medicines. *Current Problems* No. 21, January 1988.

14 Aserinsky E, Kleitman N. Regularly occurring periods of eye motility, and concomitant phenomena during sleep. *Science* 1953;**118**:273–4.

15 Williams R L, Karacan, I, Hursch C J. *EEG of human sleep: clinical applications*. New York: Wiley, 1974.

16 Brezinova, V. The number and duration of the episodes of the various EEG stages in young and older people. *Electroencephalography and clinical neurophysiology* 1975;**39**:273–8.

17 Roffwarg H P, Muzio J N, Dement W C. Ontogenetic development of the human sleep-dream cycle. *Science* 1966;**152**:604–19.

18 Morgan K. *Sleep and ageing: a research-based guide to sleep in later life*. London: Croom Helm, 1987.

19 Zepelin H, McDonald C S, Zammit, G K. Effects of age on auditory awakening thresholds. *Journal of Gerontology* 1984;**39**:294–300.

20 Monroe L J. Psychological and physiological differences between good and poor sleepers. *Journal of Abnormal Psychology* 1967;**72**:255–64.

21 Adam K, Tomeny M, Oswald I. Physiological and psychological differences between good and poor sleepers. *Journal of Psychiatric Research* 1986; **20**:301–16.

22 Morgan K, Dallosso H M, Arie T, Byrne E J, Jones R, Waite J. Mental health and psychological wellbeing among the old and the very old living at home. *British Journal of Psychiatry* 1987;**150**:801–7.

23 Morgan K, Dallosso H, Ebrahim S, Arie T, Fentem P H. Characteristics of subjective insomnia among the elderly living at home. *Age and Ageing* 1988; **17**:1–7.

24 Morgan K, Healey D W, Healey P J. Factors influencing subjective insomnia in old age: a follow-up study of good and poor sleepers aged 65–74. *Age and Ageing* (in press).

DISCUSSION

Professor Crisp Could you comment on your use of the term subjective insomnia? I understand insomnia to be a complaint about insufficient sleep.

Dr Morgan My concept of insomnia is a complaint of poor quality sleep, as perceived by the individual. There is not a direct relationship between these complaints and objective parameters of sleep. So we cannot say that insomnia means insufficient sleep or less sleep than those who do not complain about their sleep. Clinically patients' complaints about sleep are usually taken at face value without further investigation to quantify their sleep.

Audience What amount of time do the elderly spend sleeping in the 24 hours, including nodding off during the day? Surely the quality of life does influence how one sleeps?

Dr Morgan Daytime napping is fascinating. Looking at 24 hour sleep recordings in retired individuals, there is little evidence of complete compensation for lost night time sleep during the day. In people living a relatively active life, if their naps are taken into consideration they do not appear to sleep as long as they otherwise would. By lifestyle, I mean things that people do. I agree that if you live an alert and active life, this helps to maintain a sleep/wake schedule. In retirement the imposed regime of work is removed and no clear distinction may exist between leisure, rest and active periods. Sleep/wake schedules can be grossly disturbed in people who excessively nap during the day.

Audience Could you comment on the use of tryptophan in the elderly?

Dr Morgan I do not subscribe to the idea that the first line of response to a complaint about sleep is pharmacological intervention. This is a practical problem and sometimes expectations are out of line with reality. First responses should be: inculcating good sleep hygiene measures, encouraging people to get the most out of their sleep and sleep environment, and removing factors that obviously disturb their sleep. Clinical trials may show a particular compound to be harmless, but it is unlikely to have been conducted over the timespan that elderly people take sleep medication for.

Professor Crisp Tryptophan is a naturally occurring substance and is not toxic in the amounts recommended; unfortunately the evidence that it helps sleep is tenuous.

SLEEP DISORDERS IN CHILDHOOD AND ADOLESCENCE

Dr P. Hill

Senior Lecturer in Child and
Adolescent Psychiatry
St George's Hospital Medical School
London

MATURATIONAL CHANGES

Total amount of sleep

The total amount of sleep in 24 hours falls in a gentle exponential curve from birth throughout life. Although the newborn will spend some 16.5 hours asleep, a four-year-old will be asleep for only 11.5 hours and a sixteen-year-old will sleep for 8.5 hours in each full day.

Organisation of the sleep-wake cycle

A newly born infant will divide his sleep up into several spells which soon differentiate into a main sleep period and about four naps. By six months, this will have simplified into about 11 hours of night-time sleep and typically two naps, one in the morning and one in the afternoon. The morning nap tends to be abandoned by about eighteen months though the afternoon nap persists until the age of four or so. By school entry, sleep has become consolidated into a single night-time period (Figure 1).

Structure of sleep states

Sleep in the neonate can be differentiated roughly into 'active' and 'quiet' types, corresponding to REM sleep and non-REM sleep respectively. This distinction is quite clear by eight months, by which time an alternating, cycling pattern of non-REM and REM sleep is well-defined.

The electrophysiological changes within quiet sleep show progressive differentiation. By two months, sleep spindles have appeared, allowing the identification of stage 2 sleep. The first k-complexes are seen at six months and high voltage slow delta waves can be seen at about nine months. By the age of 2, sleep has acquired the basic structure seen in adulthood (Table 1).

Throughout childhood and adolescence there is a shift in the ratio of REM to non-REM sleep. The premature baby spends about 80% of sleep in REM sleep, which falls to around 50% by term. By the age of three years, this proportion will have fallen to 33%, and by puberty only 25% of sleep will be REM sleep; a figure similar to the 20% characteristic of young adult sleep

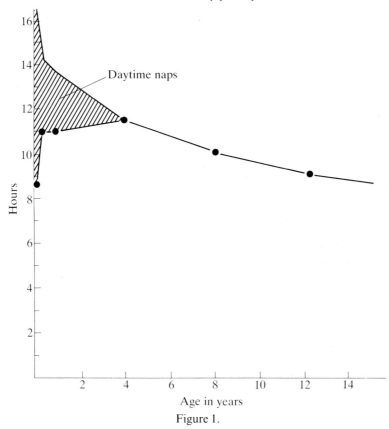

Total sleep per day

Daytime naps

Hours

Age in years

Figure 1.

(Table 2). Although a newborn baby often starts a sleep period by entering directly into active or REM sleep, this immature pattern will have been displaced by three months of age when sleep will begin by a phase of non-REM or quiet sleep.

Within the first period of non-REM sleep, there are changes with age. After the first few months of life, pre-school children start a period of sleep with a

TABLE 1. Development of sleep state

Neonate	Active (REM)
	Quiet (N-REM)
2 months	Sleep spindles
6 months	First K complexes
9 months	Phasic slow δ
2 years	Well established sleep structure

21

TABLE 2. REM/N-REM Sleep Balance

	REM sleep as percentage of total sleep time
Premature infant	80%
Term infant	50%
3 years	33%
Puberty	25%
Adult	20%

very rapid descent into slow-wave sleep, particularly stage 4 which is achieved within some ten minutes of falling asleep. They are then self-evidently very difficult to rouse, and can be moved from one room to another, or taken from a car, undressed, and put to bed without waking. There is thus a large amount of slow-wave sleep in the first three or four hours of sleep.

With increasing age, a more gradual initial descent through sleep stages into stage 4 develops, and the first period of REM sleep is more substantial. The subsequent second cycle of stage 4 sleep is of shorter duration than the first. These episodes of stage 4 sleep early in the night slowly shorten with age and are only partially compensated for by an increase in the amount of the lighter stage 3. There is a general decline in the amount of slow-wave sleep throughout childhood and adolescence, with almost all of this being accounted for by changes in the first cycle.

Parasomniac behaviour

At about 60 minutes after a preschool child falls asleep there is a sudden termination of stage 4. The result is often a partial arousal. The child can typically be seen to stir, rub his face and make a few chewing movements, subsequently turning over in bed without waking fully. He may also open his eyes briefly, even sit up but without making a fuss, so that parents are often unaware that sleep has been interrupted. Such behaviours are normal and do not cause problems. The parasomnias (sleep-talking, calm or agitated sleep-walking, thrashing and rolling, or night terrors) are in behavioural terms exaggerations and distortions of these brief partial arousals, and have an EEG configuration of mixed waking and sleep patterns.

Waking

The newborn baby cannot sustain sleep for more than a few hours. Infants and preschool children are likely to wake during the night; the more so if they are excited or otherwise aroused. Infra-red video recording shows that 85% of two month old children wake during the night; at 9 months this is 67%.[1] Such waking will most probably occur after the first REM sleep period; the child moves around the bed, rearranges bedclothes and goes back to sleep. His actions are purposive, unlike those of the parasomniac state.

Later in the night, particularly in the last third, brief wakings from light sleep are more likely.

A clinical problem produced by nocturnal waking is generally estimated to have a prevalence among pre-school children of 10–20%. There is a developmental trend, with 20% of 1–2 year-olds being affected. Only 14% of 3-year-olds wake at least three times a week.[2] These figures suggest that not all children who wake disturb their parents. Presumably a clinical problem arises out of the interplay between two groups of factors: those which cause waking, and those which represent reasons for the child being unable to fall asleep again without parental involvement.

This leads us to a list of factors shown to be associated with night waking as a clinical problem[3,4]:

- High levels of arousal
- Selective neurological immaturity
- Breast feeding
- Separation anxiety
- Parental over-responsiveness
- Too much to drink

Settling

Children have to learn to fall asleep at a socially appropriate time. This is facilitated by drowsiness, calmness, a bedtime routine to provide cues, and the presence of a parent to diminish separation anxiety and fears of the dark if these develop. However, the ultimate goal is to learn how to fall asleep in the absence of an attachment figure. Failure to achieve this is not uncommon, and presents as a clinical problem having a developmental trend affecting about 15% of 3–4 year-olds and 10% of 8-year-olds.[2] Once again, there is a list of associated factors:

- Displaced sleep–wake cycle
- Lack of routine
- Overwhelming separation anxiety
- Excessive fears of the dark
- Inadvertent or stress-related stimulation causing arousal

Adolescence

There is surprisingly little change in sleep architecture during puberty. Rather, there is a continuation of the changes which accompany and represent development: less slow-wave sleep overall, less stage 4 in particular, and shorter total sleep time. Wakings are progressively fewer, and there are less REM/non-REM sleep cycles; with the total falling from about 7 pre-pubertally to 4 or so in early adult life.

Two features of adolescent sleep are notable. One is the appearance of mid-afternoon drowsiness. This is not a phenomenon detected in normal pre-pubertal children but apparent in adolescents even when adequate sleep is allowed at night[5]. It has nothing to do with heavy lunches. The other feature is difficulty in rousing in the morning. It is not clear whether this is also evident if there has been adequate night-time sleep. In general, adolescents are likely to be chronically sleep-deprived[6] and will take opportunities to catch up on lost sleep. Part of the reason for this is the fact that evenings are times for social activities, which may be arousing by their nature, or accompanied by excessive consumption of stimulants such as tea and coffee. Interwoven with this is the tendency, when parental supervision or timetable demands are lessened (at week-ends and holidays), to revert to a 25 hour cycle, staying up later and later in the evenings so that their sleep-wake cycle is delayed. It becomes impossible to separate cultural from biological influences in shaping adolescent sleep patterns.

CLINICAL PROBLEMS I: DIFFICULTY IN SETTLING AT NIGHT

This is a common clinical problem of preschool children, with a prevalence in the order of 10–20%. Although apparently trivial, the stress on parents is severe, not least because they are exposed to a vast quantity of advice; most of it being useless. Everyone appears to be an expert, but the problem persists. Although there are a multiplicity of causes (Figure 2), these can readily be managed according to the diagram in Figure 3.

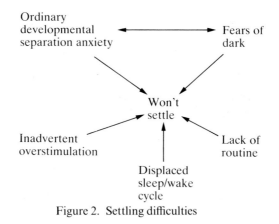

Figure 2. Settling difficulties

To start with, one should see both parents if at all possible, and tell them that:
- this is a common problem, not usually a sign of bad parenting or a spoilt child

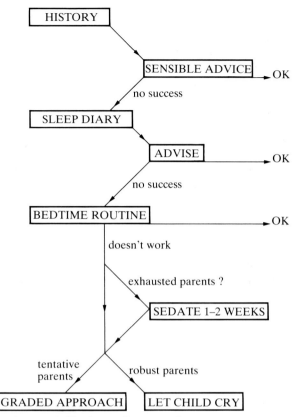

Figure 3. Difficulty settling: overall management

- it is not always that easy to deal with; there are no guaranteed short cuts
- even adults find it difficult to fall asleep by effort of will
- their first duty is to survive, not to win a battle

A small child who just will not go to sleep at the expected time may be:
1. not tired because he has had too long a sleep in the afternoon
2. not tired because he has been over-stimulated or excited just before bed
3. not tired because he customarily sleeps late in the morning (mother lets him sleep in because he got off to sleep late the previous night). Thus his sleep period is displaced later than usual but is of normal duration so that he is getting an adequate amount of sleep and is not tired at the early evening bedtime
4. frightened of being left alone or abandoned (normal separation anxiety)
5. anxious because of noises in the dark, parents having a row downstairs, or because he knows he will eventually make his mother angry

25

6. confused as to what is required of him (mother puts him to bed before father gets home, but he knows father is pleased to see him when he gets in; different bedtimes every night etc.)

The first step, therefore, is to obtain a good account of the problem—what exactly happens and why is it a problem for the parents (lack of privacy, tiredness, losing a power struggle, criticism from grandparents, lack of support from father . . .); one may be able to give sensible advice.

Next is to extend this and establish what the child's *sleep pattern* is. This may lead to the giving of sensible advice straightaway. However, as parental accounts are not always clear, it is nearly always sensible to ask the mother to keep a prospective sleep diary over the next week. This should include:

1. time awake in the morning (and whether waking was needed)
2. mood on waking
3. times and duration of naps during day
4. what time he is told he must go to bed
5. what time he is known to be asleep
6. whether he wakes during the night (time, duration and parental action)

Other details may be included (but can be omitted in most cases) such as
● what time he is taken upstairs
● which parent takes charge
● how they prepare him for bed (baths, stories, warnings, drinks etc.)
● whether/when he calls out or comes down

The diary can be drawn up on a sheet of paper (see Figure 4) and is best kept near the child's bed. One should explain to the mother what it is one wants, by drawing up columns and headings or by having a prepared sheet.

This may establish something that one can give sensible advice about:
● unreasonable parental expectations
● too much sleep during the day (think about getting him into a playgroup) but note that a *brief* early afternoon nap can improve the quality of night-time sleep
● erratic bedtimes
● displaced sleep cycle

It is wise to set a bedtime (saving repeated ill-tempered negotiations each night) and establish a bedtime ritual, with a fixed progression of events—from a warning that bedtime is approaching, through taking the child to his bedroom, undressing him, bath, tucking up, story, kissing goodnight and so on. This enables a small child who cannot tell the time to be 'cued in' to the approach of bedtime. The number of calls for glasses of milk etc. should be limited in advance. The bedroom must be congenial and enhance falling asleep (nightlight etc.). **The essential task is for the parents to help the child to learn how to fall asleep on his own.** Either setting a bedtime with routine is sufficient, or further measures are needed. If the latter, one should pause for thought.

WEEK BEGINNING	time awake	mood on waking	daytime naps (give times)	time told to go to bed	time in bed	time asleep	waking in night (give times)
Monday							
Tuesday							
Wednesday							
Thursday							
Friday							
Saturday							
Sunday							

Figure 4. Sleep diary

If the parents are at their wits' end and exhausted, then consider medication for the child for one week. Trimeprazine tartrate as Vallergan Forte syrup in a dose of *at least 60 mg* about *two hours* before bedtime usually works, though the child may be irritable the following morning for a few days initially. It may take several nights to get the dose and timing right, but a maximum of 2 weeks is a good rule for sedating a small child. One should make sure that the parents continue to use the 5 ml plastic spoon issued; domestic teaspoons can hold as little as 1.5 ml, with consequent disappointing results.

Once the parents are feeling braver, one can discuss two options with them;
1. letting him cry
2. managing things gradually

Letting the child cry is quick if the parents can manage it. Many parents will say they have tried it and it does not work. Closer questioning reveals that they could not stand the screams and gave up too soon.

Firstly ensure that the environment is conducive to sleep. A soft light (night-light or landing light), toys in the bed (not exciting ones), and a tape recorder playing a story all help.

The following steps are necessary:

1. both parents must agree with each other that they are going to do this properly (there is no dishonour in feeling it to be too brutal).
2. they *must explain* to the child what is going to happen: that, once he has been kissed goodnight, they are not going to come in to him when he cries, and that they want him to lie quietly in his bed and wait until he falls asleep.
3. the child should not be able to get out of the door, but should be able to reassure himself that the parents are still around and have not deserted him. A burglar chain on the door or a stairgate in the doorway are useful ploys.
4. the parents need to let the child know that they are still around; they should be urged to talk, sing, wash up noisily or have the radio or TV on. This is in contrast to the usual parental practice of creeping around silently 'to let him get to sleep'.
5. the parents must have something to do besides listening to the screams or they will not be able to stand it.
6. they may also have to warn the neighbours.
7. the total duration of crying before sleep should be recorded on a chart.
8. both parents must understand that the crying *gets worse at first*. Like all behaviours intended to attract, or perpetuated by, social attention crying will initially intensify and last longer if attention is withdrawn. If the parents can last out for the first 4 nights, the crying should then gradually subside. The record kept (see 7. above) will show this more clearly than the recollections of a fraught and somewhat guilty parent.
9. next morning the child can be praised for going to sleep on his own. He can stick a star on a chart or a bead on a string at the foot of his bed.

Managing things gradually (graded approach) takes longer but is more acceptable to many parents. The core programme is as follows, but may require some preparatory work if the situation is out of hand (see below)

Attend to points 1, 2 and 4 (possibly 5 and 6) as above; i.e. parents agree the procedure, tell the child, and have a contingency plan for when the child screams.

(i) The parent (mother for the sake of this illustration) settles the child briefly, *without letting him fall asleep* and leaves the room, telling him she will return in 5 minutes. The bedroom door is left ajar.

(ii) she does not return for 5 minutes unless the child gets out of bed, in which case she returns him to bed and tells him that she will shut the bedroom door if he gets out of bed again.

TABLE 3. Shutting the door on a child who gets out of bed (time door held in minutes)

Day	First Time	Second	Third and Subsequent
1	1	2	3
2	2	4	6
3	3	5	7
4	5	7	10
5	7	10	15
6	10	15	20
7	15	20	25

TABLE 4. Helping a child fall asleep alone

How long to wait before going in to child (in minutes)

Day	First time	Second time	Third and subsequent times
1	5	10	15
2	10	15	20
3	15	20	25
4	20	25	30
5	25	30	35
6	30	35	40
7	35	40	45

(iii) at 5 minutes she returns to the child and settles him briefly (about 2 minutes) and then leaves the room again. She must leave the room *before he falls asleep.*
(iv) 10 minutes later she returns and settles him briefly again.
 (v) 15 minutes later she visits once more and subsequently visits at 15 minute intervals until the child is asleep. She must always leave the room before the child falls asleep, since the object of the exercise is to help the child to learn how to fall asleep on his own. All she has to do is quieten him.
(vi) The child getting out of bed after the first warning is dealt with by the parent taking him back to bed, and then going out of the door and holding it closed for a full minute. She can talk through the door to the child, telling him that if he goes back to bed, he can have the door left open. This can be repeated as often as necessary, increasing gradually the time the door is held closed (see Table 3). Talking through the door

29

is allowed. Once he has returned to bed, at least 5 minutes should elapse before the parent returns to settle him.

(vii) After the first night, the time intervals are subsequently increased by 5 minutes each night, i.e., for the second night, 10 minutes to the first settle, then 15, then 20 (see Table 4).[7]

Similarly then if the child gets out of bed the time that the door is held shut is lengthened progressively (see Table 3.)

Most children will be settling well by the end of a week. Nearly always, the problem has resolved before getting to the 45 minute timings.

PREPARATORY WORK

Some parents will have virtually lost control of the situation and be spending enormous amounts of time in the child's bedroom. If the child is used to a parent sitting by (or lying on) the bed or cot, then one should start the training from there.

Get the parents to take alternate nights on duty to share the burden. They must stop lying on the bed next to their child and move to sitting on the edge, then, over a period of evenings, to a chair by the bed, then moving the chair each evening nearer the door until eventually they are outside the door. They should have something to do other than watch the child: reading, knitting, crosswords, even listening to a personal hi-fi. If they have been singing the child to sleep for hours, get them to hum increasingly softly each evening. The principle is *very gradual change*.

Some children, mainly the 3-year-olds and over, can be encouraged by a simple *incentive scheme*. A string tied to the bed or hung next to it can be used to store beads or buttons earned for completing certain tasks. These must start with the possible; for instance, with the child getting into bed himself, once he is dressed in pyjamas. When that has been established for a week, a new task is set and different colour beads are earned for the next stage, such as by lying down while a story is read. Then a new colour is given for lying quietly while mother goes downstairs for three minutes, and so on, each stage worked upon until it has been established for at least a week. This scheme can, of course, be used in conjunction with the graded approach programme outlined above.

If the problem concerns the child coming out of the bedroom after he has been well settled, then the child can be rewarded for going no further than the top of the stairs, then to the bedroom doorway, then for doing this without calling out, and so forth. The ultimate aim is to have the child lying peacefully in bed, prepared for sleep, staying there for an adequate amount of time and without a parent in the room.

CLINICAL PROBLEMS II. WAKING AT NIGHT (Figure 5)

As explained earlier, most small children wake during the night, but only some make a fuss about it. There tends to be an association with difficulties in

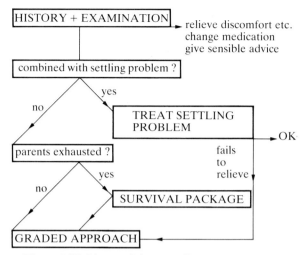

Figure 5. Waking at night: overall management

settling because the child who cannot get to sleep in the evening without a parent present will have the same difficulty when he wakes in the night. In such a case, treat the evening settling difficulty first. A variant of this is that the child may be able to fall asleep at bedtime with the landing light on, the television easily heard and with traffic outside. In the middle of the night it is dark and silent, with different conditions prevailing. It may, therefore, pay to duplicate these at bedtime (no lights, no noise from downstairs etc.).

The child who settles comfortably in the evening, yet wakes and cries in his own room (or comes into his parents' room) at night, should be examined to exclude a physical cause for discomfort: eczema, asthma, otitis media, glue ear (often overlooked as a cause of night-time discomfort), teething etc. The possibility of medication (especially bronchodilators) as a cause of insomnia should be reviewed. Other obvious problems such as noisy neighbours (or parents), or recent stress, may enable sensible advice to be given.

Some parents of frequent wakers will be too exhausted, and the nights too cold to implement a treatment programme straightaway. For such reasons the following advice (survival package) seems realistic as a medium-term measure over several weeks:

1. Parents agree to take alternate nights on duty (saves the arguments and point-scoring about whose turn it is); the child cannot insist upon the other parent dealing with him.
2. If initial attempts to soothe the child, or return him to bed fail, then the parents can be given licence to take him into their bed.
3. For the rest of the night, the parent not on duty moves out into any spare room or bed available.

31

4. If the child manages to stay in his own bed throughout the night without crying, he is praised accordingly in the morning. He can earn stars for being found in his own bed in the morning.

Medication (trimeprazine 60 mg at bedtime) can be added to take the edge off things, but should only be used as a short-term measure (1–2 weeks) to allow parents to overcome their own sleep-deprivation. Earlier studies which suggested that this drug was ineffective have been overtaken by the findings by Simonoff and Stores[8] that a dose of 45–60 mg provides reasonable (though not complete) respite.

The risks of taking a small child into the parents' bed have been exaggerated. It is an extremely common practice and in most instances has no long-term sequelae. Taking the child into the parents' bed at the beginning of the night is a different matter, because it interferes with their sex life. But this argument does not necessarily hold for the child who is taken in or allowed in during the night. Parents sometimes fear (or are told) that they will never get him out again, but in real life this does not seem to be a problem, particularly if the child is constantly reminded that staying all night in one's own bed is a sign of growing up. The cost is that the child will never learn to get back to sleep alone in the night, particularly if the nights are cold. The orthodox advice for managing children who come into their parents' bed at night is to return them straightaway and wait outside the door, calmly returning them to bed each time they emerge. However, this is arduous and may have to be repeated 20–30 times a night. Because of this, parents who are ready to deal more definitively with the problem of a waking or wandering child should apply the graded approach programme detailed above, complete with the door-closing sanction. They return the child or go in to him and settle him briefly, returning after an initial 5 minute period, which is lengthened gradually. It may be wise for the parents to arrange a strict alternate nights rota, to avoid arguments.

A child who wakes early (4–6 a.m.) is difficult to manage. Sedation often will not work. If he wanders alone around the house at such a time and thereby puts himself at risk, then the best that can be done is to ensure that there is an adequate supply of toys in his room, and keep him there with a stair-gate in the doorway. If the problem is that he comes in to the parents too early, then putting a time-switch on a bedside night-light can be helpful. If set for a suitable time in the morning it provides the child with a visual indicator of when it is appropriate to come in to the parents. This can be linked with returning him if it is too early and, conversely, praise (perhaps with stars on a chart) for not disturbing them.

CLINICAL PROBLEMS III: NIGHTMARES AND NIGHT TERRORS

Nightmares are bad dreams and occur during REM sleep. The child may cry out or wake, in which case he is clearly frightened and clingy. The contents of the dream can usually be recalled at the time or in the morning. Nightmares are common, particularly between the ages of 5 and 10 years, and do not require

32

any attention unless they are more frequent than once a week (as a rough rule), or unless there is a strong repetitive theme indicating a morbid preoccupation. It is possible to suppress them with a tricyclic antidepressant such as amitriptyline or clomipramine (not trimipramine which does not suppress REM sleep), but this treatment is hardly ever necessary. Generally speaking, preoccupations that are frightening enough to dominate ordinary dream content, producing essentially the same nightmare over a period of weeks, merit psychiatric referral.

The exception is recurrent nightmares following an identifiable traumatic experience such as an assault or serious accident. In which case, one should try combining amitriptyline 50 mg at night for one month, with attempts during the day to get the child both to talk to a parent or other trusted adult about the incident in question, and to play imaginative games or draw pictures related to it. Some theories claim that dreams assist the accommodation of daytime experiences in memory. This raises the question as to whether it is sensible to suppress dreams with medication. Formal studies of REM sleep deprivation do not demonstrate any harm arising from dream suppression, and, whilst it is wise not to meddle unnecessarily with sleep, a short course of a tricyclic antidepressant can free the child from avoidable terror.

Night-terrors are an instance of so-called parasomnias which arise out of one of the first phases of very deep (stage 4) non-REM sleep; in other words, before midnight and often about 1–3 hours after falling asleep. The parents hear a shriek or loud burst of crying and run to the child, who is found sitting up in bed or stumbling around the bedroom with open eyes. They may notice a racing pulse, dilated pupils and tremor; signs of a very high level of psychophysiological arousal. The child may appear hallucinated, fending off invisible attackers with his hands, and may call out briefly to them. He will push his parents away and not cling to them. It is impossible to get through to him in spite of his appearing awake. After a few minutes he returns to sleep and has no memory for the episode in the morning.

Such attacks are much commoner than most textbooks imply, although, no formal prevalence figures have been established. They seem to be particularly likely in children under 5, though can occur at any age. It used to be said that they indicated deep psychological disturbance, but there is no evidence for this in pre-school children. However their frequency will increase if the child is stressed. There is no justification for the assertion that they reflect a disturbance in the parents' sex life, though given the timing of a typical night-terror, it can certainly disrupt it. The myth persists because the sex life of many parents of young children is likely to be at an unsatisfactory stage, for a number of understandable reasons.

The appropriate course to take with night-terrors is

1. to reassure the parents. They should be told that the phenomenon is a disturbance of sleep which the child will grow out of. They should not try to wake the child during a terror.

2. to keep a prospective record of recurrent night terrors, so as to identify the time at which they are most likely to occur. Once this is established, the

parents should fully wake the child 15 minutes before the projected time each night for a week, subsequently allowing him to go back to sleep after 2–3 minutes (anticipatory waking)[9]. This often abolishes the problem by encouraging the development of a different pattern of sleep stages. Often and with good effect, it can be extended to the treatment of other parasomnias (see below).

In the unusual instance of excessive frequency (e.g. more than one night in three for one month) and resistance to the above method, then night terrors can be abolished with diazepam 2–6 mg given at bedtime (benzodiazepines reduce stage 4 sleep). Although it might seem logical to use a short-acting benzodiazepine, this can merely postpone the terror to the final hours of the child's sleep, which is even more disruptive to parents' sleep. Continue for three weeks, then discontinue gradually.

CLINICAL PROBLEMS IV: SLEEPTALKING, SLEEPWALKING, THRASHING IN BED AND TOOTHGRINDING

Normal pre-school children are likely to show brief movements such as face rubbing, squirming, muttering or moaning, and abrupt sitting up in bed about 1–2 hours after settling. These occur for a few seconds as the child emerges sharply from the first phase of very deep (stage 4) sleep. If pronounced or prolonged they are called parasomnias. These phenomena arise out of a disturbance in the integration of the stages of sleep, and are not the result of disturbing dreams. All are common and typical of older, mainly school-age, children. Usually there is a family history. They can be listed on a scale of increasing severity (Table 5).

TABLE 5. Parasomnia spectrum

Severe	Full blown night panic
	Night terror
	Confused thrashing + moaning
	Agitated sleepwalking
	Calm sleepwalking
	Sitting up in bed with blank expression
	Sleeptalking
	Eye opening
	Mumbling
	Chewing
	Rubs face
Mild	Turns over

Sleeptalking rarely requires medical intervention beyond reassurance. It can be suppressed by anticipatory waking (if regular in its timing), or a benzodiazepine, but this is hardly ever necessary.

34

Sleepwalking is potentially dangerous; there is no truth in the adage that sleepwalkers come to no harm. The parents must ensure that the bedroom windows are secure, and must consider putting a gate across the child's doorway. It may be wise to move the child to the lower bunk bed where this applies. Older children may manage to reach the front or back door, and these will then have to be locked or bolted with a high bolt.

There is no point in waking a sleepwalking child; they will have no memory for the episode in the morning. Although they are obviously confused whilst walking, they are not basically psychologically disturbed. The best course of action is nearly always to steer them back to bed gently, playing the whole thing down, and ensuring that the child is safe. If there is a regular pattern, then waking the child 15 minutes before a likely episode each night, for a week, as for night terrors, will usually work. If absolutely necessary, benzodiazepine suppression of slow wave sleep can be implemented (see p. 34). This may be necessary if the disorientated, sleep-walking child is prone to urinate in cupboards, or if night terrors and sleep-walking combine so that the child rushes around the house in a confused panic. Even so, it is wise to obtain a prospective record in case a pattern can be established and anticipatory waking tried first.

Some children *thrash* around in bed in a confused, inaccessible state which may occasionally go on for several minutes. They lack the apparent fear of a night terror but usually respond to a week of anticipatory waking.

Toothgrinding in sleep (bruxism) seems likely also to be a parasomnia. The usual empirical remedy, however, is dothiepin 50–75 mg at night rather than a benzodiazepine. If severe and protracted, a dental opinion may be necessary to check for enamel damage.

CLINICAL PROBLEMS V: NIGHT ROCKING, BANGING AND HEADROLLING

A number of ordinary small children develop rhythmic habits, which seem to help them get off to sleep. These include sitting up and rocking backwards and forwards or side-to-side. They are harmless, even when quite alarming head-banging is involved, and nearly all children have abandoned the practice by the age of 4. The appropriate intervention is reassurance and practical measures to minimise noise (padding cot sides, putting foam under the cot legs). It may occasionally be possible to set a metronome to match the frequency of rocking, and then gradually slow it, night by night, starting it off as the child settles to sleep.

CLINICAL PROBLEMS VI: INSOMNIA IN ADOLESCENCE

The causes of insomnia in adolescence are much the same as those in adult life (Table 6). The complaint of insomnia by the adolescent, rather than by the parents, usually means trouble getting off to sleep or poor quality sleep with frequent waking. Parental complaints are usually about late bedtimes, which may well be compensated for by late rising, so that the adolescent is

TABLE 6. Insomnia in adolescence

Anxiety
Depression
Licit/illicit medication
Recent drastic dieting
Coexistent physical disorder
Head injury

---

actually getting adequate sleep. If this is out of hand, try putting them on a 27 hour day, so that they go to bed an hour later each night until they work round to a normal bedtime again. Most adolescents with insomnia have other psychological abnormalities, especially mood disorders, which may be primary, but are more likely to be secondary to stressors. This means it is necessary to enquire about anxiety, depression, life events and life circumstances.

It is wise to ask about all medication, licit and illicit, though an adolescent who is abusing drugs which prevent sleep (amphetamines or anticholinergics) is unlikely to complain of poor sleep himself. Cola drinks, coffee and tea intake, appetite suppressants should all be asked about specifically. Recent drastic dieting may itself unsettle sleep.

The management of adolescent insomnia is unlikely to involve hypnotics as a first line, unless there has been a recent and short-lived stress. More usually there should be an attempt to seek underlying causes of psychological distress, with simple advice to the adolescent to avoid lying in bed trying fruitlessly to sleep. Rather, he should get up and read in another room, returning to bed only when drowsy. Tuition in relaxation is a useful adjunct, and it is sensible to advise minimal daytime sleep. A hot milk-based drink at bedtime is as effective as the advertising claims and not to be dismissed.

CLINICAL PROBLEMS VII: ADOLESCENT HYPERSOMNIA

Hypersomnia as perceived by parents may actually be paralleled by the teenager complaining of poor quality sleep, as in sleep apnoea and narcolepsy (Table 7). Both are discussed elsewhere in this booklet.

Most adolescents who are difficult to wake in the morning have gone to bed too late, or are just normal people who are not at their best in the morning. A very few will prove extraordinarily difficult to wake and act aggressively if attempts persist. Some of these will have so-called hypersomnia with sleep drunkenness[10]. This is an obscure but very real disorder in which the adolescent sleeps long hours, is hard to rouse, is ataxic and irritable for an hour or so when woken, and may be considerably disadvantaged, particularly when moving away from home to college or the armed services.

TABLE 7. Excessive daytime sleepiness
in adolescence

Narcolepsy
Sleep apnoea
Hypersomnia with sleep drunkenness
Kleine-Levin syndrome
(Substance abuse)

Kleine-Levin syndrome[11] is an extremely rare disorder but important to bear in mind. In this condition, which appears only to affect boys, there is periodic hypersomnia so that the patient leads an ordinary life for several months in between bouts. In a bout he is assailed by irresistible light sleep with clouding of consciousness so that most of each day is spent asleep. When awake, the boy gorges food, raiding the fridge and snatching food from other people's plates at mealtimes. His weight will increase so rapidly that vivid abdominal striae can be seen. Whilst asleep he is likely to experience lurid dreamlike fantasies with a sadistic or sexual content. A typical episode lasts several days, perhaps a couple of weeks, and will repeat several times a year. There are anecdotal reports of the effectiveness of lithium prohylaxis (with which I can concur), though the expectation is that the condition burns out in early adult life.

REFERENCES

1 Anders T. Home recorded sleep in 2- and 9-month-old infants. *Journal of the American Academy of Child Psychiatry* 1978;**17**:421–32.
2 Richman N, Stevenson J, Graham P. *Preschool to School.* London: Academic Press, 1982.
3 Anders T. Neurophysiological studies of sleep in infants and children. *Journal of Child Psychology and Psychiatry* 1982;**23**:75–83.
4 Eaton-Evans J, Dugdale A E. Sleep Patterns in infants in the first year of life. *Archives of Disease in Childhood* 1988;**63**:647–49.
5 Carskadon M. Determinants of daytime sleepiness; adolescent development, extended and restricted sleep. Ph.D. Thesis. Stanford University, Stanford, California, 1979.
6 Webb W, Agnew H. Are we chronically sleep deprived? *Bulletin of the Psychonomic Society* 1975;**6**:47–8.
7 Ferber R. *Solve Your Child's Sleep Problems.* London: Dorling Kindersley, 1985.
8 Simonoff E, Stores G. Controlled trial of trimeprazine tartrate for night waking. *Archives of Disease in Childhood* 1987;**62**:253–57.
9 Lask B. Novel and non-toxic treatment for night terrors. *British Medical Journal* 1988;**297**:592.
10 Roth B, Nevsimalova S, Rechtschaffen A. Hypersomnia with sleep drunkenness. *Archives of General Psychiatry* 1972;**26**:456–62.
11 Orlosky M. The Kleine-Levin syndrome: a review. *Psychosomatics* 1982;**23**:609–21.

DISCUSSION

Audience   Could you comment on hyperactivity in relation to sleep disorders?

Dr Hill   A parental complaint of hyperactivity often means disobedience until proved otherwise! There are conflicting reports about real hyperactive children; one is that they sleep soundly and cannot be aroused, the other is that hyperactive children hardly sleep at all. My impression is that there is no association with any sleep disorder, but I know of no study that has explored this.

Audience   I understood that sleep changes in depression present as a tendency to oversleep in the younger patient, but you did not discuss this as a cause of hypersomnolence in adolescents. What are your views?

Dr Hill   There are only two studies of adolescent depression that have considered sleep. In both those studies oversleeping was more common than undersleeping, but sleep disturbances and sleep duration were not common features of adolescent depression[1,2]. In my clinical experience, sleep disruption is not commonly complained of by adolescents who are clinically depressed.

Audience   What is your management of children who headbang during sleep?

Dr Hill   Head-banging, head-rolling, leg-rolling are all common in small children's apparent efforts to get to sleep. 5% of pre-school children show vigorous rhythmic motor behaviour getting off to sleep. Perhaps head-banging during the night is performed by children who have woken up and are getting back to sleep. It is a not uncommon clinical problem; the most common pictures are either a child that sits up against the cot bars and bangs his head backwards against them, or the child who gets onto all fours and rocks forward and bashes his head against the top of the bed. The child seems to be neither fully awake nor fully asleep when doing this. It is terminated by sleep and appears to be associated with very light sleep or the initial phase of going off to sleep. The management ought to be explanation and reassurance given to the parents. I know of no instance of a child damaging himself by this form of head banging. It is less severe and less frequent than the head banging indulged in by the seriously mentally handicapped or autistic. One management strategy that appears to help is the use of a metronome in the bedroom. The parents set the tick to the frequency of the head-banging and then gradually slow it every night, but I only have data for this intervention on three children. Strong rhythmic behaviours in small children going off to sleep seems to be quite common, but they become uncommon in children over three.

Audience   The Americans consider night-time rocking to be a non-REM sleep dysomnia. I would agree with you that head-banging in the average child does not appear to cause damage; American studies of full medical examination and X-rays of these children after prolonged banging show no sign of any damage.

Professor Crisp I am suspicious of the Kleine-Levin syndrome in terms of the suggestion that it is an organic syndrome; although the effects of brain damage could possibly lead to that behaviour. MacDonald Critchley, described one or two cases in male adolescents of hyperphagia and hyper-somnia[3]. In an eating disorder clinic there are adolescent males with bulimia nervosa who would fit into this pattern of episodic behaviour with episodic bingeing and loss of control. It has been recognised that patients can eat themselves into somnolence, and patients with eating disorders can adopt this as a defensive strategy against loss of control. Retrospectively such episodes may be seen as episodes of encephalitis, which have spawned a subsequent eating disorder, but I consider them to be functionally determined. Under these circumstances sexual fantasies would not be unusual, because the problem is one of impulse control generally. Do you think your two cases might have fallen into that category?

Dr Hill I think they are radically different; the history from one patient is remarkably clear. He describes the first manifestation as a feeling of unreality and of the world slowing. This persists for one or two days, then he starts to feel drowsy. Over the next two days he descends into extreme sleepiness, so that sleepiness and the fantasies are well established before the eating starts. The eating is easy to control environmentally, just by clearing the house of food. He is disinhibited, and will walk around the house masturbating. In his account there is a gap of several days between the onset of an altered mental state and the eating. Another way of managing the eating is to use fenfluramine in high doses—80 to 120 milligrams a day—during a phase. This may control overeating, but it does not appear to affect the somnolence which does not respond to stimulants either.

REFERENCES

1 Hudgens R. *Psychiatric Disorders in Adolescents.* Baltimore: Williams and Wilkins. 1974.
2 Inamdar S, Siomopoulos G, Osborn M and Bianchi, E. Phenomenology associated with depressed moods in adolescence. *American Journal of Psychiatry* **136**:156–59.
3 Critchley M. Periodic hypersomnia and megaphagia in adolescent males. *Brain* 1962;**85**:627–57.

NARCOLEPSY AND THE HYPERSOMNIAS

Dr J D Parkes
Reader in Neurology
Institute of Psychiatry, London

By narcolepsy I mean the specific illness, the narcoleptic syndrome. Patients with daytime drowsiness fall into four categories. The commonest is the narcoleptic syndrome, the second is obstructive sleep apnoea, the third is probably drowsiness post glandular fever, persisting for many years, and the fourth is totally undiagnosable by me.

NARCOLEPSY

Firstly a look at the clinical features; secondly, a look at the fascinating genetic and environmental factors in narcolepsy (which have emerged as one of the most interesting stories in medicine in the last few years); and then a few general points.

The French neuropsychiatrist, Gelineau, is credited with the first description of the illness; he was of equal distinction for his work in psychiatry on agoraphobia. This led him to separate the fear of an agoraphobic patient crossing a Parisian square and being driven over by a carriage from the collapse with laughter of patients with catoplexy-narcolepsy. He described this illness as 'seizing with sleep'. The narcoleptic syndrome is a serious illness, with daytime drowsiness causing considerable disability. Sometimes these patients are wrongly diagnosed for many years before narcolepsy is recognised, they may be accused of amphetamine addiction or malingering.

Black patients with narcolepsy have been highlighted in recent years because of the genetics of the illness. One of the first black subjects described in the American literature was a courageous slave from the southern states who helped others to escape in the early civil war, Harriet Trubman. She had unequivocal narcolepsy and possibly cataplexy described in the 1800's.

CLINICAL FEATURES

The diagnostic feature is of persistently going to sleep under unusual circumstances. This is the cardinal symptom required to make a diagnosis of daytime drowsiness in the narcoleptic syndrome. This must be coupled with one of two other features: either cataplexy, as determined by the clinical history or unequivocal frequent sleep paralysis occurring many times a year, to make the diagnosis.

TRIGGERS OF CATAPLEXY

The trigger is usually a sudden increase in alertness due to excitement, surprise, many sports, e.g., a good shot at tennis, catching a fish. Laughter is a common precipitant. Clinical diagnosis requires a trigger followed by two features—firstly paralysis, and secondly loss of muscle tone.

SLEEP PARALYSIS

Sleep paralysis is terrifying, and may lead to ritualistic behaviour. Sleep paralysis is the equivalent of REM sleep atonia accompanied by self-awareness. Hypnagogic hallucinations (pre sleep dreams) are a misnomer; they are the equivalent of REM sleep dreams whilst the subject is awake. The subject gives a history of dreaming before being asleep, or dreams in the daytime when he or she is not asleep. (This is not usually a helpful feature diagnostically.) People have looked for an autonomic defect but the evidence is not clear. Two features sometimes observed during REM sleep, loss of tendon reflexes, corresponding to what happens during sleep atonia, together with an extensor plantar response, but these are not invariable. Patients with cataplexy may fall down and break bones, but cataplexy is probably less frightening than sleep paralysis. However, cataplexy can be even more disabling than narcolepsy in patients who have frequent episodes.

The seminal discovery that went a long way to explain the physiology and pathophysiology of narcolepsy was the finding by Rechtschaffen and his colleagues of early onset REM sleep in this illness.[1] In the narcoleptic syndrome one is seeing a dissociation of sleep and dreams that occur during REM sleep from the mechanisms of motor control.

A variety of structural lesions have been described in the narcoleptic syndrome. The latest has been demonstrated on nuclear magnetic resonance scanning and will probably prove to be artefactual; no pathological lesion has ever been found in any patient with unequivocal narcolepsy cataplexy. A variety of CSF studies have provided no meaningful answers to date.[2] Neurotransmitters in the sleep systems remain totally unknown.

EPIDEMIOLOGY

What of the epidemiology of the narcoleptic syndrome? The incidence of the condition appears to vary enormously from country to country, although reliable figures are lacking. The reported figures show a prevalence range from 0.2 through 16 per 10 000. According to one report only six patients with narcolepsy have been identified in Israel compared to a high prevalence in Japan. There is no accurate estimate for the UK but a guess is that there are 20 000 people with narcolepsy in the UK, in other words it is a common illness. Attempts have been made to correlate these findings with the incidence of HLA DR2, which has 99.5% linkage to the narcoleptic syndrome.[3] There is some evidence that the incidence of narcolepsy follows the incidence of DR2 in different populations.

There is a familial basis to narcolepsy. About a third of patients with narcolepsy have a history of a first degree relative with similar illness; the pattern of inheritance is almost certainly autosomal dominant.[4] Genetic studies indicate that if a disease shows autosomal dominant inheritance, there is probably a single coding defect for a cell surface protein molecule; so the hunt is on to find this single coding defect in narcolepsy. Once this has been elucidated it is hoped that the way will be open to investigate sleep neurotransmitters and sleep mechanisms at the molecular level.

Amazingly 99.5% of people with narcolepsy have on the surface of their lymphocytes the HLA antigen DR2 but a few do not. The gene coding for DR2 is almost certainly not the narcolepsy gene.

Many illnesses have been described in association with the narcoleptic syndrome (Table 1). Two of the most interesting are multiple sclerosis, and the post encephalitic group. Diabetes is interesting in that patients with Type I diabetes lack DR2. So possibly DR2, as seen in narcoleptic syndrome, acts as a protective factor against diabetes.

TABLE 1. Associated diseases
Association between 'narcolepsy' and other diseases

Disease associated with narcolepsy	Notes
Possible immune mechanisms	
Polycythemia	Occasional association with
Lymphoma	narcolepsy, but very uncommon
Systemic lupus erythematosus	in all instances
Disseminated sclerosis	
Pernicious anemia	
Probable sleep apnoea, not narcolepsy	
Acromegaly	Probably always sleep apnoea
Myotonic dystrophy	
Dysautonomias	
Ocular disorders	
Extrinsic muscle paralysis	?Embryonic defect
Cataract	
Glaucoma	
Metabolic disorders	
Diabetes mellitus	Not true narcolepsy. DR2+ve
Thyroid disease	rare in type 1 diabetes mellitus
Miscellaneous	
Essential tremor	(Single patient only)
Parkinsonism	(Two patients)

From: Parkes *et al.*: In: Honda Y, Juji T (eds) *HLA in Narcolepsy* 1988: 165.

A report from Czechoslovakia and Germany has demonstrated that every patient considered to have post encephalitic narcolepsy or post encephalitic sleep disorder is DR2 positive.[5] This is a remarkable observation which may suggest that the encephalitis lethargica virus or a related virus can trigger a true narcoleptic syndrome in these patients.

There is an unequivocal relationship between multiple sclerosis (M.S.) and narcolepsy. This is not due to the demyelination itself. The narcoleptic syndrome may precede M.S. by 20 years or more, it may be severe, yet the patient has no symptoms of multiple sclerosis for many years then develops optic atrophy, or tingling of a limb, for example. More detailed studies of what gene codes for a DR2 molecule in these two illnesses have revealed a specific epitope of DR2 in both disorders.

Twin studies highlight features of environmental and genetic factors in illness. There are reports of monozygous twins discordant for the narcoleptic syndrome.[6] Assuming that the monozygous twins have absolutely identical genetic makeup, this would suggest a major environmental contribution as well as genetic. Narcolepsy demonstrates the strongest HLA association of any disease followed by rare forms of pemphigoid skin disorders, and then by ankylosing spondylitis.

ANIMAL MODELS

Animals models of narcolepsy exist and are being intensively investigated. There are dogs from Stamford which get narcolepsy, and Shetland ponies which get a form of narcolepsy which differs in few ways from the human version.

SUSCEPTIBILITY TO CLINICAL MANIFESTATION

Possibly narcolepsy, like myasthenia gravis, is an immune mediated disease.[2] Unfortunately there is little evidence to support this view. It has been reported that many patients with the narcoleptic syndrome have high anti-streptolysin titres (ASO) but this finding requires confirmation.

It is easy to speculate about possible sleep neurotransmitters that may be involved in narcolepsy, but there are little meaningful data. The gene coding for vasoactive intestinal peptide (VIP) is on the same chromosome –6– as the HLA systems, but the two are a considerable distance apart. Interestingly, the human suprachiasmatic nucleus, a controller of the 24 hour biological clock, is full of VIP. Venoms from a particular group of sea snails cause sleep and are used to paralyse prey, causing a behavioural and electrical picture of sleep in the victim. Researchers are using these conus geographicus toxins to explore the nature of sleep and of the narcoleptic syndrome.

TREATMENT

Established treatment is with dexamphetamine, methyl phenidate or mazindol. We start narcoleptics on mazindol 1–2 mg once or twice a day.

Eldepryl is interconverted to methamphetamine and amphetamine thereby having a stimulant effect. Whether its stimulant effect in narcolepsy is entirely due to this or to MAOB inhibition is unknown. In doses exceeding 30 milligrams a day it begins to inhibit MAOA, as well as MOAB, and so is potentially dangerous in these high doses. There is no totally pure MAOA or B inhibitor, but this treatment appears to be useful in a dosage of 5 or 10 milligrams a day for people with the narcoleptic syndrome.

Imipramine is a successful treatment for cataplexy, but of any drug, clomipramine has the most specific effect on cataplexy. Within 24–48 hours of starting clomipramine 10–25 mg/24 hours, cataplexy is abolished. On withdrawing the clomipramine a rebound of cataplexy is seen within 2 or 3 days. This may be temporarily worse than the starting point.

DIAGNOSIS

Firstly, the diagnosis is founded on clinical and historical evidence; an occasional amphetamine addict who is sophisticated may mislead the clinician with a convincing history. Secondly, for practical purposes the patient must be HLA DR2 positive. If he is HLA DR2 negative then he probably has not got narcolepsy. The exceptions are in the black population; only 60% of black subjects with the narcoleptic syndrome are HLA–DR2 positive.

SLEEP STUDIES IN NARCOLEPSY

EEG sleep studies—are they of any value? They are expensive and time consuming. Most clinicians in the UK do not have access to sleep laboratories run by experts. A request for 'EEG, query narcolepsy' is meaningless. Evidence of early onset REM sleep within the first 10 minutes of going to sleep is found in patients with narcolepsy, but a single negative EEG is totally unhelpful. Conditions other than the narcoleptic syndrome can cause early onset REM sleep; sleep deprivation itself or normal pattern of entry into sleep in infancy. Repeated EEGs performed in a good laboratory, may be useful, but as a solitary screening procedure an EEG is of little value.

REFERENCES

1 Rechtschaffen A, Wolpert E A, Dement W C. Nocturnal sleep of narcoleptics. *Electroenceph Clin Neurophysiol* 1963;**15**:599–609.
2 Parkes J D, Langdon N, Lock C B. Narcolepsy and immunity (editorial). *Brit Med J* (clin res) 1986;**292**(6517): 359–60.
3 Honda Y Juji T (eds). *HLA in Narcolepsy*. Springer Verlag Berlin, 1988:208.
4 Baraitser M, Parkes J D. Genetic study of narcoleptic syndrome. *J Med Genet* 1978; **15** (4): 254–9.
5 Andreas-Zietz A *et al*. DR2 negative narcolepsy (letter). *Lancet.* 1986;**ii** (8508):684–5.
6 Montplaisir J, Poirier G. Narcolepsy in monozygotic twins and non-genetic factors in narcolepsy. *5th International Congress of Sleep Research*, Copenhagen, Denmark. 1987:401.

DISCUSSION

Prof Crisp   In my experience clomipramine appears to block hypotonia during REM sleep. Would Dr Parkes care to comment?

Dr Parkes   The whole field of sleep atonia is a marvellous mystery. Why are muscle tone and reflexes lost? What is the mechanism? One model is that there is a pathway in the brainstem firing onto the anterior horn cell and inhibiting it. If a healthy subject is put to bed and his REM recorded and then his central conduction time measured to see what is happening at the anterior horn cell level, there does not seem to be inhibition at the anterior horn cell by a descending pathway. At present this is a fascinating area of physiology but with no answers. Dr Horne, what are your views on why we lose motor tone?

Dr Horne   Dr Adrian Morrison, from the University of Pennsylvania has been exploring a motor inhibitory centre in the locus cerelleus which produces hypotonia in REM sleep.[1] If this centre is destroyed, then normal motor responses occur, and the animal moves about during REM sleep, apparently acting out its dreams. This would be a dangerous state of affairs for the animal, and hence, a paralysis has to be induced by the brain during REM sleep.

Dr Parkes   I do not believe that these animal studies can be extrapolated to men. There are half a dozen rare brain stem diseases, from progressive supranuclear palsy upwards and downwards, destroying the locus cerelleus in humans, which do not seem to have any behavioural effect. Many of the studies of physiology we are basing our ideas of sleep on are from cats, dogs and rats, with very different sleep patterns from human beings. Perhaps sleep has different functions in these animals from ourselves.

Dr Horne   There are the rare humans who do not have motor inhibition in REM sleep and flail around whilst asleep. I think that the important point is that with us there has to be some active inhibition of the motor response in REM sleep to keep us immobile, otherwise we would endanger ourselves and everybody else.

REFERENCE

1 Morrison A. A window on the sleeping brain. *Scientific American* 1983;**248**:86–94.

SLEEP APNOEA AND SNORING

Dr J Stradling
Honorary Consultant Physician
Osler Chest Unit, Churchill Hospital, Oxford

Before we can understand how sleep affects breathing, let us briefly recap the basic control mechanisms of respiration.

PHYSIOLOGY

The respiratory muscles include the diaphragm, the intercostal muscles and the important upper airway muscles. The upper airway is a floppy tube which would collapse on inspiration without the upper airway muscles to maintain patency. All these muscles are controlled via the spinal cord and the brain stem centres. The most important drive to respiration is unconscious, coming from the brain stem—the CO_2 drive, and indirectly the hypoxic drive. This is always operative, but can be overriden by higher centres, for example when talking. When sleeping, particularly during slow wave sleep, this higher centre control is lost and only the metabolic controls of respiration remain. This is a major difference between wakefulness and sleep.

In slow wave sleep, respiration is very regular (Figure 1). The size of the breaths, the speed of the breath and the frequency of the breaths are all very regular during slow wave sleep, when the metabolic control of respiration is dominant.

In rapid eye movement sleep, the phase when we dream most, breathing becomes irregular, with drop outs and cessations of breathing which are entirely normal (Figure 1). This is believed to be due to influences outside the respiratory centre, more similar to wakefulness again. '

When in slow wave sleep, most breathing is done with the rib cage indicating intercostal muscle activity and very little by the diaphragm (reflected in the abdominal contribution). On passing into rapid eye movement (REM) sleep the abdominal contribution increases because the intercostal muscles suffer from a normal physiological inhibition during REM sleep. We are truly paralysed during REM sleep apart from the diaphragm. This paralysis therefore also includes the upper airway muscles.

These changes in the way respiration is brought about during sleep lead to certain points of vulnerability in its control, allowing disorders of respiration to occur, thus leading to nocturnal hypoxemia. During non-REM sleep (or slow wave sleep, which is the deeper phase of non-REM sleep) there is a fall in overall respiratory drive because of the removal of the awake cerebral component already referred to. This leads to a reduced output to the diaphragm, and the other respiratory muscles. This includes the

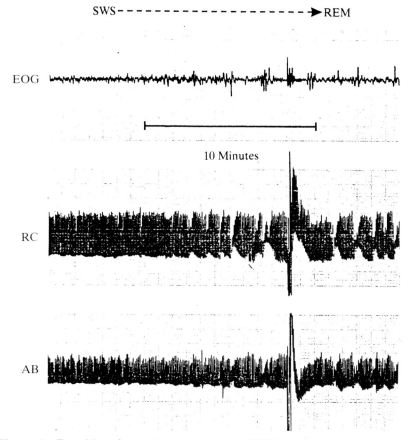

Figure 1. Transition from slow wave sleep (SWS) to rapid eye movement sleep (REM) showing the change in ribcage (RC) and abdominal (AB) excursion. Note that as the eye movements (EOG) of REM come in, the breathing becomes irregular.

muscles in the upper airway, so that upper airway resistance increases and may provoke snoring. During REM sleep there is a further loss of this muscle tone and, from studies using EMG electrodes inserted into the upper airway muscles, we can demonstrate almost a complete dropout of EMG tone. Thus, the diaphragm is the only muscle left working which may be a serious situation if this muscle's function is impaired. There is a fall in the functional residual capacity of the lungs because of loss of intercostal muscle tone, which may increase $\mathring{V}/\mathring{Q}$ mismatching in people with pre-existing lung disease. In addition, when you are in dreaming sleep, compared with slow wave sleep, much greater stimuli are required to wake you, so more hypoxia and hypercapnia can be tolerated before arousal and restoration of breathing.

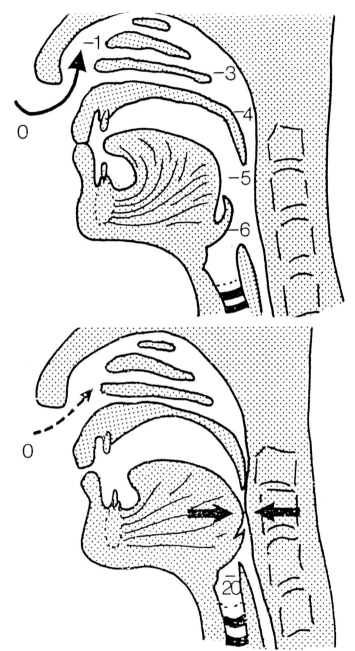

Figure 2. Diagrammatic representation of upper airway collapse in obstructive sleep apnoea (see text).

SLEEP APNOEA SYNDROMES

Rigid definitions of sleep and breathing disorders are probably inappropriate. Sleep apnoea should be regarded as important only if the cessation or diminution of breathing during sleep leads either to arousal or hypoxemia. We all have episodes of stopping breathing during sleep, but if they do not lead to hypoxemia or arousal, they are harmless. A syndrome is present if there are sufficient numbers of events to cause symptoms during the day. In the most common condition, obstructive sleep apnoea, the upper airway collapses on going to sleep, leading to repeated obstructed inspiration. The other non-obstructive sleep and breathing disorders are a heterogeneous group, usually due to failure of respiratory drive, which only occur rarely. These conditions tend to present mainly with the consequences of sleep disruption, and far less commonly with diurnal respiratory failure.

Obstructive sleep apnoea is simple to understand; on breathing in, the pressure in the upper airway becomes subatmospheric because of resistance to airflow in the nose (from the turbinates). The upper airway tends to collapse unless it is adequately supported which leads to a simple passive collapse (Figure 2). Obstructive sleep apnoea is simply a failure to maintain the patency of the upper airway on falling asleep. Early on in the apnoeic phase the respiratory efforts are small because there is little respiratory drive but as the CO_2 rises and the oxygen falls, the respiratory effort increases against the blocked pharynx. The brain will say, 'Hang on, you've got to do something about this,' and the subject will wake up with an explosive snorting and snoring, clear the upper airways, and return the blood gases to normal. That arousal is not usually enough for the patient to be aware of it, so he will not present complaining of waking up many times every night as one might expect. Unfortunately this destroys the quality of the sleep, so the individual does not get stage 3/4, high quality, restorative slow wave sleep. The severely affected patient may be unable to sleep and breath at the same time, having in the order of 300 apnoeas per night. If the oxygen saturation is recorded overnight via a finger oximeter, normal subjects would rarely drop below 95% during sleep (Figure 3a). Subjects with obstructive sleep apnoea show dips in oxygen saturation when they become apnoeic and then the levels rise again as they rouse themselves (Figure 3b). The number of arousals can be counted from the oximeter tracing and there may be as many as 350 on this tracing.

FACTORS DETERMINING UPPER AIRWAY COLLAPSE DURING SLEEP

Why do some people have this problem with a collapsed upper airway and others not? The upper airway is a floppy tube which is compliant, and without suitable support forces it will collapse. The subatmospheric intrapharyngeal pressures when breathing in are believed to play an important role in this condition (Figure 2). If there is a high upstream resistance, such as with a partially blocked nose, the walls are sucked in more and hence collapse is more

49

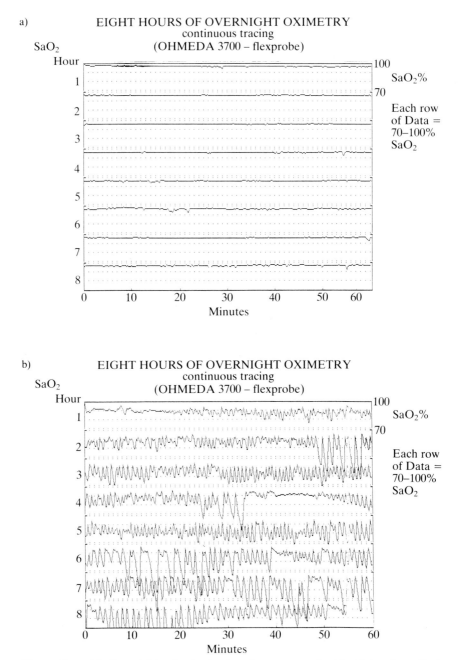

a)

EIGHT HOURS OF OVERNIGHT OXIMETRY
continuous tracing
(OHMEDA 3700 – flexprobe)

SaO₂
Hour

SaO₂%

Each row
of Data =
70–100%
SaO₂

Minutes

b)

EIGHT HOURS OF OVERNIGHT OXIMETRY
continuous tracing
(OHMEDA 3700 – flexprobe)

SaO₂
Hour

SaO₂%

Each row
of Data =
70–100%
SaO₂

Minutes

Figures 3a and b. Overnight oximeter tracings from a normal subject (a) and a patient with obstructive sleep apnoea (b).

likely. People snore more readily when they have a blocked nose and this is merely a 'forme fruste' of obstructive sleep apnoea. If the pharynx is small initially it will collapse more readily. In addition, the muscles responsible for holding open the upper airway may be important in this condition.

ANATOMICAL OR MUSCLE FAILURE?

There are many case reports of this condition associated with structural abnormalities of the upper airway such as acromegaly, large tonsils, mucopolysaccharidoses, SVC obstruction, lymphomas and carcinomas in the upper airway. In any condition that narrows the upper airway behind the tongue, a patent airway can be maintained whilst awake, but when the normal loss of muscle tone is superimposed at night this leads to collapse. There is also an association with obesity, specifically obesity in the neck[1] due to the compressive force of the mass weight of fat. Using sophisticated methods to measure the volume of the upper airway lumen it has been demonstrated that people with sleep apnoea have small volume upper airways. The structure of the jaw may be subtly different in these people, not necessarily obviously receding jaws as in Pierre Robin syndrome, but a subtle variation in normality. The evidence for high upstream resistance and small starting size is over-whelming, but there are those people who believe that the muscle power is also important. It is certainly important when considering the effects of drugs and

Figure 4. Overnight oximeter tracings on a control night and after moderate alcohol consumption in a heavy snorer (from Issa and Sullivan, 1982)[2]

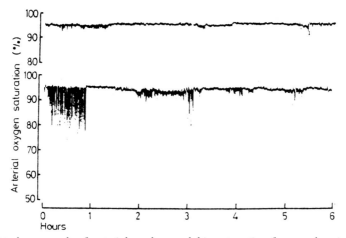

All-night slow records of arterial oxyhaemoglobin saturation from a chronic snorer. A, control night; B, alcohol night. Although continuous snoring occurred on the control night, there were no episodes of obstructive apnoea and no oxyhaemoglobin desaturation. Note the repetitive episodes of desaturation in the first hour of sleep following alcohol; these resulted from obstructive apnoeas.

alcohol on the upper airway. The overnight oxygen saturation tracings in Figure 4[2] demonstrate the effects of alcohol in somebody who is a heavy snorer but had a reasonably good night's sleep. Before the second tracing, the subject had the equivalent of 1 to 2 martinis and developed marked obstructive sleep apnoea in the early part of the night. From clinical and laboratory based experiments alcohol is a potent inhibitor of the upper airway muscles, hence many people will snore after alcohol and not otherwise[2]. As the tracing shows, the effect passed off during the course of the night as the alcohol level fell.

My conclusions about sleep apnoea are that the causes of obstructive sleep apnoea are largely due to anatomical problems, but poor pharyngeal muscle tone can contribute, particularly when alcohol, sedatives, or (as recently shown) sleep deprivation are superimposed.

The sort of symptoms patients present with are legion (Table 1). Patients are referred from a bewildering variety of sources, from the neurologists, general practitioners, psychiatrists as well as self-referrals. Most of these patients will snore heavily but when they finally present, the snoring may have diminished because they either breathe when they are awake, or do not breathe when they are asleep, and the interim phase is so short that they hardly snore. But a history of snoring is almost 100%. Virtually all these patients will complain of being sleepy, and this is the most serious symptom. For the individual who cannot work or concentrate because he is sleepy, life can be absolute hell. Many of these people have lost jobs, they have lost marriages, and are in a

TABLE 1. Range of symptoms, grouped by frequency, experienced by patients with sleep apnoea

---

Common (> 60%)
        Loud snoring
        Excessive daytime sleepiness
        Choking or shortness of breath feelings at night
        Restless sleep
        Unrefreshing sleep
        Changes in personality
        Nocturia

Less common (10–60%)
        Morning headaches
        Enuresis
        Reduced libido
        Spouse worried by apnoeic pauses
        Nocturnal sweating

Rarely (< 10%)
        Recurrent arousals/insomnia
        Nocturnal cough
        Symptomatic oesophageal reflux

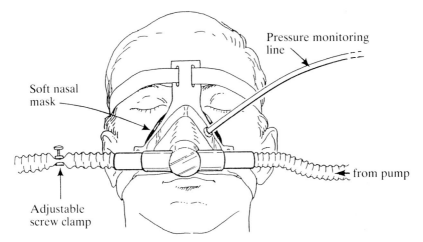

Pressure monitoring line

Soft nasal mask

from pump

Adjustable screw clamp

Figure 5. Equipment used to treat obstructive sleep apnoea—nasal continuous positive airway pressure–CPAP.

sorry state. Some would prefer to be dead than sleep their lives away. Patients may record that they have sleep disturbance, but most think they have a good night's sleep. The incidence of car accidents in this group is very much higher than normal: in one USA state, it is calculated to be about seven times normal[4].

TREATMENT

Simple first line therapy consists of no alcohol after 6 p.m., no sedatives, to sleep on the side—to avoid the jaw weight effect, to keep the nose clear, to lose weight, and to stop smoking. However, if a patient is severely affected, treatment with continuous nasal positive airway pressure may help (Figure 5). The theory behind this treatment is that if the upper airway is collapsing, why not blow it open during sleep? This is done by a fan pump blowing air under pressure via a nose mask. It converts an abnormal overnight oximeter tracing to normal (Figure 6).

There are surgical treatments available, but the selection criteria for patients who will benefit have not been identified. The most commonly used procedure is a uvulo-palato-pharyngo-plasty, really only for a patient who has a big soft palate and preferably large tonsils, to try and create a bigger upper airway.

CHILDREN AND SLEEP APNOEA

The ENT unit in Oxford has a particular interest in sleep apnoea in children. In children with obstructive sleep apnoea, the pattern is rather different from adults. It is highly irregular varying with sleep state and body position. An

53

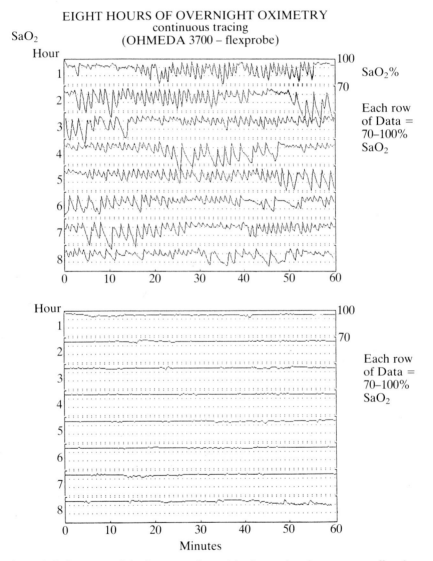

EIGHT HOURS OF OVERNIGHT OXIMETRY
continuous tracing
(OHMEDA 3700 – flexprobe)

SaO₂

Figure 6. Oximeter tracings from a patient with obstructive sleep apnoea off and on nasal CPAP therapy.

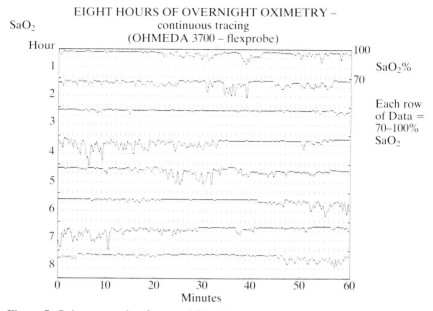

Figure 7. Oximeter tracing from a child with obstructive sleep apnoea due to large tonsils.

oxygen tracing would look like that in Figure 7 with periods of irregular obstruction when the child falls asleep. Compare this tracing with Figure 3b.

About 70 of these children who had been referred to the ENT department with large tonsils, who also snored, have now been studied. Their oxygen saturation dip rates per hour were measured. Over 5 dips per hour were taken to be abnormal. Over one-third of these children have an increased amount of nocturnal hypoxemia and after tonsillectomy the levels return to the normal range (Figure 8). In trying to measure what this might do to these children, weight centiles were measured before and after tonsillectomy (Figure 9). There was a 20% rise in weight centiles which is significant. Of course the rise in weight may not be due to the removal of the sleep disturbance, it might simply be that they no longer have a sore throat and can eat better. Height centiles are less likely to be affected in this way (Figure 9) and an average 13% significant rise in height centiles was noted after tonsillectomy. This is considered to be an important indicator that something was wrong with these children before their tonsillectomy. Growth hormone is released during slow wave sleep and we know these children do not get enough slow wave sleep due to their sleep fragmentation. Interestingly some of these children did not have hypoxemia, but on video recordings had obvious sleep disturbance. To actually measure this a technique was developed to measure movement of the child. Using the all-night video recordings that we now make, during video playback, movement is logged and then expressed as a percentage of time spent moving. Most

Dips/hr of SaO$_2$ (>4%) before and after tonsillectomy

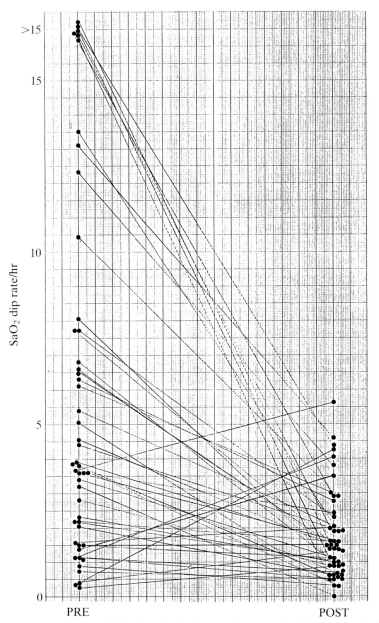

Figure 8. Frequency of 4% dips in SaO$_2$ per hour in 48 children booked for tonsillectomy, pre and post surgery.

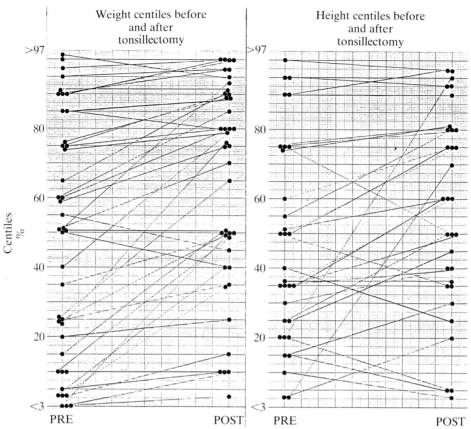

Figure 9. Change in weight and height centiles following tonsillectomy in children.

of the children studied with this system had increased percent time spent moving which returned to normal range after tonsillectomy. So even when there is no hypoxemia on the oximeter, these children are having disturbed sleep.

In conclusion sleep apnoea appears to be common in children with large tonsils who snore. Presumably most children grow out of it as their tonsils atrophy, but there will be a period when they have sleep disturbance. In a very few this can become severe enough to lead to respiratory failure. I strongly suspect that there are important interferences with the child's growth and development.

CONCLUSIONS

Sleep apnoea is an important, interesting and easy to understand condition. It affects adults, and is probably more common than we are aware of. In children something as common as enlarged tonsils and snoring may be contributing to retarded growth and development. Unless we remember to consider sleep and breathing disorders, we will miss the opportunity to help a large number of patients.

REFERENCES

1 Stradling J R, Warley A, Mitchell J. Correlates of nocturnal hypoxaemic dipping in normal men aged 35–65 years. *Europ Resp J* 1988; in press.
2 Issa F G, Sullivan C E. Alcohol, snoring and sleep apnoea. *Journal of Neurology, Neurosurgery and Psychiatry* 1982;**45**:353–9.
3 Bonora M, Shields G I, Knuth S L, Bartlett D, St. John W M. Selective depression by ethanol of upper airway respiratory motor activity in cats. *Am Rev Respir Dis* 1984;**130**:156–61.
4 Findley L J, Uverzagt M E, Suratt P M. Automobile crashes in patients with obstructive sleep apnoea. *Sleep Research* 1988;**17**:178.

GENERAL ARTICLES

1 Guilleminault, C, Tilkian A, Dement C. The sleep apnoea syndromes. *Ann Rev Med 1976;***27**:465–84.
2 Guilleminault W C, Korobkin R, Winkle R. A review of 50 children with obstructive sleep apnoea syndrome. *Lung* 1981;**159**:275–87.

DISCUSSION

Dr Horne   I wonder if Dr Stradling could elaborate on the impact of benzodiazepines on sleep apnoea?

Dr Stradling   It is really the same as alcohol. There are some good experiments from Monique Bonora in the States that look at the respiratory output to the diaphragm and compare it with the respiratory output to the upper airway muscles. Agents such as benzodiazepines, barbiturates, any of the anaesthetic agents and alcohol, all depress the upper airway long before they affect the respiratory drive to the diaphragm. Hence giving benzodiazepines for poor sleep seems to be disastrous.

Audience   Dr Stradling, some authorities suggest that 100% of children with sleep apnoea have enuresis. What causal mechanism is suggested? Does this give any possible openings in terms of treatment for refractory childhood enuretics?

Dr Stradling   Personally I do not agree with that 100% figure which was quoted from Gemineau's original description. I believe it to be secondary enuresis recurring. In the sleep apnoeic children seen in our unit only 10% have had a return of enuresis. Conversely in recalcitrant enuretics this mechanism should be sought. Perhaps this is why tricyclic antidepressants sometimes work in enuresis, by altering the amount of REM sleep, which would be increased as a rebound phenomenon from the sleep deprivation. I do not understand why children with obstructive sleep apnoea are enuretic, perhaps they are so sleepy they just do not wake up when they feel like going for a pee.

Professor Crisp   There is a suggestion that nocturnal enuresis occurs most often in transition between sleep stages, particularly 4 and 3. Although with obstructive sleep apnoea patients do not get to 4 very often, when they do they quickly move back up to 3 or 2, exhibiting a lot of movement between sleep stages.

Dr Stradling   One of the diagnostic criteria for sleep fragmentation in these people is the number of sleep state changes. This is a powerful index of how disturbed the sleep state is.

Audience   Dr Stradling, what forms of drug therapy do you use in adults with sleep apnoea?

Dr Stradling   There was quite a vogue for two forms of drug therapy. Firstly, the tricyclic antidepressants where the mode of action is not entirely clear. There are two possible explanations. One is that obstructive sleep apnoea is worse during REM sleep because of the greater inhibition of the upper airway muscle tone, and if the amount of REM sleep is reduced it thereby reduces the amount of sleep fragmentation. The alternative mechanism is that the tricyclics have the opposite effect to the benzodiazepines in the upper airway muscles; there is a small effect increasing upper airway muscle tone and they have small effects on snoring and on obstructive sleep apnoea, but in anybody who is badly symptomatic they are not clinically effective. Recently there was a report from the Toronto group who did a controlled trial comparing tricyclics and nasal continuous positive airway pressure. Both seemed to have the same effect on symptoms, but unexpectedly, the tricyclic antidepressants had no effect on the sleep apnoea, suggesting that the tricyclics were dissociating the symptoms from the actual cause. The other drug possibility is progesterone. Nobody knows how that works, and it is not a powerful effect. The first suggestion was that it is mild respiratory stimulant, or it may work by redistributing fat. A female distribution of fat tends not to be in the neck. A third drug, which was used transiently, was strychnine!

Dr Morgan   Dr Stradling, could you comment on the age-related increase and its clinical relevance in sleep apnoea?

Dr Stradling   Our community survey has certainly shown that it is related to age. The Toronto group suggested that it was due to instability of respiratory control, but have been unable to show that decreasing chemoreceptor responses are in any way important. In women it is age and menopause related, which may be related to fat distribution. Another simple suggestion is that the upper airway muscles become more flabby and less able to maintain patency.

So the mechanism is not totally clear. American studies suggest that 50% of normal people over 65 fulfil their criteria for abnormal breathing during sleep! There is also a suggestion that considering morning performance in people who are mildly demented, the overnight deterioration in mental performance correlates with the amount of disturbed sleep that they get from breathing abnormalities. So if you already have some cerebral pathology and add sleep disturbance, you will be less able to perform the following morning.

FUNCTIONS OF SLEEP

J A Horne
Department of Human Sciences
Loughborough University
Loughborough
Leicestershire LE11 3TU

SUMMARY

Total sleep deprivation findings show that the organ most affected is the brain, especially the cerebrum. The rest of the body seems to cope surprisingly well, indicating little sign of stress or malfunction. Although there are claims that sleep is necessary for general body tissue growth and repair, the underlying evidence has alternative explanations. Excluding the cerebrum, tissue repair may not rely so much on sleep, but on food intake and rest.

Following sleep deprivation, only a specific part of the lost sleep is made up. This and other evidence suggest that a certain portion of sleep ('core' sleep) is essential (i.e.—for the cerebrum), and that the remainder ('optional' sleep) is more dispensable, being more under a behavioural drive to sleep.

SLEEP DEPRIVATION

Hormones

The most obvious way of finding out what the functions of sleep might be is to deprive people of sleep and see what happens. One of the most telling indices is to look at the output of various hormones. Studies on humans of up to 205 hours total sleep deprivation (TSD), without the addition of other stressors (such as food restriction, heavy exercise, and simulated battle stress) have revealed little effect on hormonal output.[1] The most recent studies on healthy subjects, where corticosteroid output over 1–2 days of TSD was carefully assessed, revealed little sign of any change,[2] adding to the large body of nil findings from previous studies. Corticosteroid output during TSD will only increase significantly if the subjects are otherwise stressed. For example, if they are apprehensive about what is going to happen. If subjects are confident that little harm will come to them, then there is little corticosteroid response. The role of psychological distress in elevating corticosteroid output is well known.

Sleep deprivation does not lead to any change in the daytime release of growth hormone, but there is a drop in the output of some sex hormones, which is not of clinical importance.[2] Twenty-four hourly levels of urinary catecholamine output stay the same. The overall conclusion from these findings with hormones is that sleep loss produces no sign of any emergency reaction, but rather, clear indications of physiological and psychological deactivation. Obvious circadian rhythms in most of these hormones are apparent, especially with melatonin, where a significant degree of covariance between this rhythm and those of body temperature and self-assessed fatigue ratings is to be found.

Metabolism

Recent experiments looking at the effects of TSD on rodents[3] point to failures in metabolism and/or thermoregulation. Animals die after about two weeks of TSD, although, it is not yet known whether these specific failures are the actual cause of death. Early during the TSD regime, the animals eat voraciously, but nevertheless, body weight still falls. Body temperature remains stable at first, but then drops. Several reports[1] have noted that human subjects report increased hunger during the first 1–2 days of TSD, particularly during early morning. Food intake is usually well in excess of that predicted for an increased energy requirement through being awake rather than asleep. Seemingly, this desire for food seems physiological rather than just a response to boredom.

The circadian rhythm in body temperature remains intact during TSD, although, there are several reports of a small downward shift in the daily average temperature, and subjects feel the cold more. This is a common finding from our laboratory, for example. But because subjects are allowed to put on more clothing, this increased heat insulation confounds any true changes to body core temperature.

The physiological ability to perform exercise is not affected by TSD.[4,5] However, endurance falls and there is a decline in the time to exhaustion. But this is due to psychological factors, which also increase the subjects' perception of the magnitude of the exercise.

In all, the findings from human studies do point to some apparently minor problems with thermoregulation and metabolism. Of course, for a relatively big mammal like us, having a large body mass and thermal capacity, any decrement in the ability to conserve heat is of far less consequence to survival than it is in the case of small mammals.

The Immune System

It is commonly thought that in 'real life', sleep loss depresses the immune response. However, the stress causing the lack of sleep (such as anxiety and overwork), rather than the sleep loss itself, seems to be the cause. Although the effects of TSD on the immune system remain little explored, there are some interesting findings. Only two studies[6,7] have been conducted, from the same laboratory. Both reported statistically significant changes in certain aspects of the immune response. But physiologically, these were small and seemingly of minor clinical importance. The earlier investigation, of three days of TSD, also incorporated simulated 'battle stress', which may have had a more substantial effect than the TSD itself. This is indicated by the raised cortisol and adrenaline outputs, which were not found in the second study where this stress was absent. Neither study looked to see if antibody production was affected.

Psychophysiological Changes

There are signs that TSD may have minor effects on the regulation of other human physiological systems, and attention has recently been paid to respiration. The breathing response to changes in blood oxygen and carbon dioxide levels seems to become depressed.[8] The extent to which this represents an impairment to the breathing control centres or just a dampening of response due to the overall decrease in arousal, is a matter which is unresolved. Many aspects of respiration are sensitive to changes in arousal, with the most obvious being yawning (no-one knows the function of yawning). Irregularity in respiration rate increases progressively up to three days of TSD, and so does cardiac irregularity,[9] but these changes are minor. No clinically significant abnormalities of respiratory or cardiac function have ever been reported for normally healthy subjects, even in the longest studies of 205 hours and 264 hours of TSD.[10,11]

Neurological Findings

Only two, somewhat dated investigations[12,13] have performed comprehensive neurological assessments on TSD subjects. The earlier one concerned the single subject from the 264 hour study, and found no neurological changes of clinical importance. The other, of five days of TSD in eleven subjects, reported that 'easily detectable abnormalities in the standard neurological examination can occur after 60 hours without sleep'. These included nystagmus, neck muscle weakness, hand tremor, and altered body movement patterns. However, such effects were not serious and there was no question of withdrawing subjects. A common finding with most sleep deprivation studies after 1–2 nights TSD is diplopia.[14]

Neither of these two neurological investigations examined higher cerebral function, but concentrated on mid-brain and brainstem mechanisms. There is overwhelming evidence from numerous other studies, using psychological tests, that higher brain functions are impaired, and that it is the cerebrum where the most obvious effects of sleep loss can be found. These are quite apparent by the second night of TSD,[15,16] and will be discussed in the next section.

EEG findings with sleep deprived subjects usually indicate changes clearly indicative of excessive sleepiness. There are increasing numbers of reports of heightened epileptic-like activity in those people with some history of epilepsy, or for whom there are already suspicions of epilepsy. But for the majority of other subjects, free of this history, TSD seems unlikely to cause such activity, although, a small proportion may be at risk when TSD progresses beyond 2–3 days. However, this conclusion is based mostly on findings from military studies, where there are other stressors in addition to TSD; there is a dearth of 'civilian' investigations in this respect. It should be remembered that elevated corticosteroid output does seem to facilitate epileptic attacks. Interestingly, one night of TSD is thought by some to be useful as an evocative procedure for diagnosis in patients with suspect seizures.[17] Such EEG abnormalities occur most commonly during drowsiness and light sleep.

Behaviour, and Psychological Performance Changes

There have been several recent reports on apparent mood improvement following one night of TSD or REM sleep deprivation in people suffering from endogenous depression, which has been the topic of excellent reviews.[18,19] It has been claimed that REM sleep deprivation may lie behind the mood enhancement.[18] This type of mood change during TSD is uncommon in normal healthy subjects, perhaps because of a 'ceiling' effect, as mood is usually already fairly good. It is rare for healthy subjects to experience symptoms of depression during TSD, although they may appear to become 'withdrawn' because of sleepiness.

TSD obviously produces increasing sleepiness and seriously impairs concentration. What is also very apparent is that within the 24 hour period, nighttime brings the worst decline and daytime a levelling off, or even some improvement, particularly around 1800–2200 hours. These circadian changes are reflected in behaviour and psychological performance tests. The daytime levelling of performance may well be the net result of a performance fall due to increasing TSD, countered by the inherent circadian rise in arousal. At night these two factors would be additive. Whilst performance is disposed to take this stepwise trend over time, the detriment is influenced substantially by the subject's attitude, and whether he/she applies increasing mental 'effort' in compensation. This can be a successful countermeasure for up to two nights of TSD, particularly if the task is inherently interesting, varied and involves perceptual-motor skills.[15] However, tasks which are simple, dull and prolonged are very sensitive to sleep loss (e.g. watching monitoring devices, motorway driving). Such activities also enhance disinterest and sleepiness. If an incentive for doing well is added to these tasks (e.g. money or competition), then the subject can apply more effort, and performance improves dramatically during short-term TSD.

In sleep deprivation research the emphasis in psychological performance measurement has been on those tests that are most sensitive to sleepiness, are easy to score, and are not prone to large practice effects that would cancel out any impairment due to sleepiness. So the preferred tests are dull, monotonous and unstimulating, such as 10–20 minutes of simple reaction time or vigilance testing. These are more inclined to assess the motivation to perform, rather than the inherent capacity to do so. But because such tests readily show significant effects of sleep loss, we cannot assume that they are also measuring behaviours fundamental to the understanding of sleep function.

Complex tests like reading comprehension, IQ performance and decision making, show little effect of total sleep loss until the second night.[1,15,20] Such tasks are absorbing and stimulate one to apply more compensatory effort to counteract the motivational decline. However, they are only tapping some aspects of performance. In providing a selection of possible answers, IQ tests involve convergent thinking, encourage the subject progressively to 'home in' on the solution, and are easily scored.

However, little is known about the effects of sleep loss on 'creative thinking', that is, on skills requiring spontaneity and flexibility. Tests of this type are difficult to score, and have largely been ignored by sleep deprivation research since the famous studies at the Walter Reed Laboratory, in the USA, carried out thirty years ago.[21] For example, their 'Cognitive Disorganisation' scale, showed that spontaneous thinking deteriorated quite rapidly during sleep deprivation. The scale is not precise, and is now seldom used.

Many TSD studies have been conducted under constant environmental conditions, which can add to the tedium and motivational decline. This is particularly evident when the TSD is repeated under the same conditions. A form of perceptual deprivation may develop which can produce visual illusions even without TSD. So, although visual illusions (e.g.—'spider on the wall', 'fog' around lamps) are common during TSD, it is not really known to what extent these are exacerbated by perceptual deprivation. Such illusions are sometimes referred to as 'hallucinations', but real hallucinations (i.e. gross distortions of the environment) are very rare, and for example, there was only one brief such occurrence amongst all the subjects of the 205 hour and 264 hour TSD studies.[10,11] There have been erroneous claims that TSD can produce 'models' of psychosis, based partly on the misconception of 'hallucination' occurring under both states. However, it should be remembered that most psychotic hallucinations are auditory, contrasting with the minor visual illusions of TSD. Both groups of investigators in the longest TSD studies reported that no psychotic-like events occurred.

Subjects may become more suggestible during TSD, and if they are led to expect visual illusions, then these events will happen more readily. Irritability is common, but very much depends on social interactions and the level of tedium during TSD. Occasionally, subjects can be quite seriously affected and may become irrational. In our experience, TSD only produces such effects in those people who tend to have this kind of behaviour anyway, under non-TSD conditions. Subjects of a sanguine disposition only suffer this problem to a minor extent, and usually remain aware of their irritability and will not deny it.

Recovery Sleep

Most of the adverse behavioural and performance effects of TSD are overcome after one recovery night of extended sleep, though there is more recovery sleep to come. When the total excess sleep over all recovery nights is added up, only about 30% of the lost sleep is regained.[1] However, this recovery sleep contains most of the lost stage 4 sleep and about 50% of the lost REM sleep.

All of the lost stages 1 and 2 sleep, which normally make up about 50% of our sleep, seem to be dispensed with. These are some of the findings which have led me to propose[1,22] that not all of our usual night's sleep is essential to the brain, and that only the first 5–6 hours sleep appear to be crucial to normal wellbeing. This sleep (**core** sleep) contains all of our nightly stage 4 sleep, and about half the REM sleep. The latter part of sleep (**optional** sleep) is more flexible, and can be reduced or extended (without affecting daytime sleepiness), depending on safety, boredom, seasonal changes in daylength, etc. Several studies have shown that we can fairly easily adapt to 1.5–2.0 hours less sleep per day.[23] The topic of core and optional sleep is discussed more fully below.

Conclusions about Human Sleep Deprivation

To date, the findings strongly indicate that for humans the major effects of TSD centre on the brain, particularly the cerebrum, with the rest of the body incurring few, if any, real problems. There are indications that the fine regulation of certain autonomic systems (e.g. thermoregulation) may be affected. But this does not seem to be of any consequence for humans. There are no reports of physical illness during or following TSD. Although the psychological and EEG effects of TSD point to malfunctions indicating that sleep serves some essential role for the cerebrum, there is still no direct evidence to show that sleep is truly restorative for the brain, i.e. that some form of repair is taking place. Instead, there may simply be an accumulation of a sleep 'substance',[1] whereby sleep has little restitutive benefit, and for example, is simply a drive behaviour for occupying the night. There are signs that at least the later part of our sleep (optional sleep) may be under this form of control.[1]

TISSUE REPAIR AND SLEEP

Main Arguments

There is a commonly accepted idea that a major role for human sleep is to promote heightened tissue repair and protein synthesis following the 'wear and tear' of wakefulness for most of the body. This theory is called the 'body restitution hypothesis' for sleep. But the findings from TSD research that I have outlined above, and have described in detail elsewhere,[1] do not endorse such a generalised restitutional function for sleep, only perhaps for the cerebrum. In fact, I argue[1] that for the majority of organs, excluding the brain, human sleep is not a state of heightened body restitution, but is more likely to be one of tissue dissolution.

The main evidence gathered in support of the body restitutive hypothesis,[24] is based on: (a) heightened cell division and protein synthesis during sleep, (b) in humans, a surge in growth hormone (hGH) output that occurs during stages 3 and 4 sleep, (c) the effects of exercise on sleep.

66

Exercise depresses cell division and protein synthesis. This has different implications for rodents and humans, in respect of whether body restitution can proceed unhindered during wakefulness. Rodents exhibit a near-continuous physical activity (exploring, foraging, grooming) during wakefulness, and for them, immobility during wakefulness hardly exists. Therefore, restitutive processes are inhibited during wakefulness due to the high levels of physical activity. As sleep is the only effective immobiliser in the rodent, these processes can only proceed unhindered then. Therefore, in these animals sleep is, by default, simply a vehicle for increased body restitution as it is the only provider of real rest. In humans and other mammals with advanced forebrains, there is the behavioural repertoire for relaxed wakefulness. We spend much of wakefulness in sitting, and in doing so, allow body restitution to proceed unhindered then.

Food intake is the main stimulus to body tissue repair.[25] In many people, the last meal of the day is completed by about 1900 hours, and the peak of tissue restitution passes by around midnight. Sleep turns into a fast, and rather than restitution, tissue degradation becomes the prevailing state (the brain might be excluded here). Breakfast, like other meals, reverses this condition.

In humans, circadian peaks in cell division often occur at night during the sleep period, and this finding has also been used in support of the body restitutive hypothesis for sleep. But such an occurrence is simply a time of day phenomenon, as it is still apparent in the small hours of the morning if the subjects remain awake.[26]

The sleep-related hGH release also seems to have been misinterpreted. Although it is commonly assumed that this release is indicative of tissue growth, there is no confirmation of this. Humans are fairly unique amongst mammals in showing such a growth hormone output, as it is absent in the majority of other mammals that have been examined in this way. One of the many functions of hGH is not only to encourage tissue growth and repair, but to help protect proteins from increased breakdown during fasting (proteins can be used as an emergency energy source) and to encourage the use of fats instead. A fasting state usually accompanies sleep in humans, and it should be remembered that for us, night-time sleep is relatively long as mammalian sleep goes; often there are 12 hours without food, from the evening meal to breakfast. In summary, the hGH release in human sleep may be protecting tissue proteins, not increasing them. Finally, sleep can override feelings of hunger at night. Poor sleepers who wake up in the night often notice how hungry they feel.

A further area which has been misleading from the viewpoint of restitution and sleep has been the effects of exercise on sleep. Stages 3 and 4 sleep (collectively referred to as slow wave sleep—SWS) may increase after daytime exercise.[27] SWS has been particularly associated with body restitution because of its connection with the hGH release. So, the SWS rise after the apparent extra muscle 'wear and tear' of exercise seemed to support the body restitution hypothesis. But it now seems that these EEG changes following exercise are associated with the body and brain temperature rise that often accompanies exercise, and has nothing to do with muscle wear and tear. If brain temperature is increased passively, for example, by the subject lying in a warm bath, then the same SWS rise is found.[28] On the other hand, if heavily exercising subjects are kept cool by cold air, to reduce the body and brain temperature increase, then there is no change in SWS.[29] Raising the brain's temperature elevates its metabolism, particularly, cerebral metabolism, and we believe that this is a more central cause of the rise in SWS. Interestingly, we have found that sustained sensory and perceptual stimulation during the daytime (which also increases cerebral metabolism), also leads to heightened SWS.

Conclusions

Although much is still unknown, there is as yet no conclusive evidence demonstrating that any organ apart from the brain (i.e. the cerebral cortex) specifically needs sleep. Physical rest and feeding may well be all that is required by the majority of tissues for restitution. Although reduced physical activity may allow a greater rate of repair, in humans similar levels of physical activity to those found in sleep can be attained during wakefulness. For example, in a subject lying relaxed but awake, skeletal muscles (excluding those of the head and neck) attain a level of tonus which is only marginally higher than that of sleep. This is also reflected in the small fall in O_2 consumption (about 8%) in sleep, compared with that of relaxed wakefulness.[30]

However, unlike the rest of the body, the cerebral cortex cannot shut down and relax to any significant degree during wakefulness. Even when we lie relaxed but awake in a quiet dark room, the cerebrum remains vigilant and in quiet readiness, prepared to respond to any stimulus and not able to demonstrate any diminution in responsiveness (i.e. 'rest'). Only during sleep, and especially during SWS, is there some release of the cerebrum from this readiness. If the brain does require some level of off-line recovery for any significant period of time, then sleep, particularly SWS, seems to be the most likely state where this could occur. The state of greatest natural cerebral shutdown in humans is SWS, especially stage 4 sleep, and as will be seen, this type of sleep seems to be essential; more so than any other sleep stage.

HOW MUCH SLEEP DO WE 'NEED'?

Core and Optional Sleep

Our daily intake of food and water is usually more than the physiological requirement, and the opportunities for most of us to eat and drink are ever present, with social customs encouraging this further. Most people can reduce their daily fluid intake by 30–50% without any consequence, as homeostatic adjustments are easily made. Whilst we cannot go to this level of reduction in food intake, a 15–20% cut in calories will, for most of us, produce no more than an initial fall in body weight that stabilises at a lower level. There is no long term harm to health. As will be seen, there are strong signs that similar notions also apply to sleep, and I argue[1] that from the perspective of sleep function, sleep can be divided into the two forms I introduced briefly earlier. That is: (i) an apparently essential component—**core** sleep, occupying about the first three sleep cycles, and centring on SWS (especially stage 4 sleep), and to some extent REM sleep; (ii) a more dispensable form—**optional** sleep, occupying the remainder of sleep.

At the onset of normal nighttime sleep, both core and optional sleep are active, with core sleep lifting after a few hours, to let optional sleep continue. Optional sleep may be some form of non-restitutive drive behaviour for occupying the remaining hours of darkness, maintaining sleep until waking-up time. Optional sleep also seems to be under the influence of a sleep-wake circadian rhythm. Nevertheless, optional sleep is flexible. Given the time for adaptation, it can be reduced or even extended further, depending on safety, boredom, and perhaps seasonal changes in daylength (in the days before artificial lighting when humans were heavily reliant on daylight). Such a core-optional division can also be applied to the sleep of other mammals[1], although here, I shall only concern myself with humans.

Evidence

Briefly, the evidence favouring this outlook comes from several experimental findings, discussed in detail elsewhere:[1]

(a) As I mentioned before, following sleep deprivation most of the lost stage 4 sleep and about half of the lost REM sleep are reclaimed. This rebound in stage 4 sleep takes priority over the partial rebound of REM sleep.

(b) During short-term reduced sleep regimes, psychological performance is not seriously impaired until, coincidentally or otherwise, SWS is restricted. That is, when sleep is below five hours duration.[31]

(c) Under long-term sleep restriction, subjects who normally sleep 7.5–8.0 hours a night can successfully adapt to 6.0 hours sleep daily, without increased daytime sleepiness.[23,32] This is achieved by the loss of the last sleep cycles—that is, at the expense of stages 1,2 and REM sleep, but not SWS. The absolute amount of SWS is maintained.

(d) After 1–2 nights without sleep, long sleepers absorb the extra demand for SWS into a recovery sleep that is no longer than normal, whereas short sleepers extend their recovery sleep to accommodate this SWS demand.[33]

(e) Natural short sleepers seem to have wholly or partly lost the usual latter part of sleep. What is left is very similar in structure (particularly in SWS and REM content) to the first sleep cycles of age-related normal length sleepers.[1]

(f) Daily sleep can be extended easily by about 2.0 hours through oversleep and daytime naps, without reducing the length of the following night's sleep.[34] Unfortunately, no long-term studies have been done here.

Arguments that the ability to oversleep implies chronic sleep deprivation[35] are debatable, and I believe[1] that this extra sleep is probably surplus, in the same way that we will often eat food, such as biscuits and cakes, just because it is available, and not because we are hungry or really need to eat.

The function of SWS is unknown. Earlier I argued that if sleep has any tissue restitutive role, then the organ that would seem to benefit the most from this would be the cerebrum. But I emphasise that we do not know whether recovery (e.g. dendritic growth and repair) of the cerebrum does occur during SWS. There are only indications that this could happen, and this may only be circumstantial evidence. These indications are: (i) cerebral neuronal firing rates are lowest during stage 4 sleep; (ii) of all the sleep stages it is SWS, particularly stage 4 sleep that correlates most positively with the length of prior wakefulness, and in this repect could fit a recovery role; (iii) increasing the brain's work (metabolism) during wakefulness, through raising brain temperature or through prolonged daytime sensory stimulation, lead to increases in SWS; REM sleep levels are unaffected; (iv) there are various studies[36] indicating that during SWS the cerebrum enters into an unique condition of isolation from both sensory input and from subcortical structures; a state that is not found in REM sleep.

REFERENCES

1 Horne J A. *Why We Sleep: The Functions of Sleep in Humans and Other Mammals.* Oxford: Oxford University Press, 1988.

2 Akerstedt T, Palmblad J, de la Torre B, Marana R, Gillberg M. Adrenocortical and gonadal steroids during sleep deprivation. *Sleep* 1980;**3**:23–30.

3 Gilliland M A, Bergmann B, Rechtschaffen A. High EEG amplitude NREM sleep deprivation in the rat. *Sleep Research* 1986;**15**:218.

4 Horne J A, Pettitt A N. Sleep deprivation and the physiological response to exercise under steady-state conditions in untrained subjects. *Sleep* 1984;**7**:168–79.

5 Martin B J, Chen H-I. Sleep loss and the sympathoadrenal response to exercise. *Medicine and Science in Sports and Exercise* 1984;**16**:56–9.

6 Palmblad J, Kantell K, Strander H *et al.* Stressor exposure and immunological response in man: interferon-producing capacity and phagocytosis. *Journal of Psychosomatic Research* 1976;**20**:193–9.

7 Palmblad J, Petrini B, Wasserman J, Akerstedt T. Lymphocyte and granulocyte reactions during sleep deprivation. *Psychosomatic Medicine* 1979;**41**:273–8.

8 Cooper K R, Phillips B A. Effect of short-term sleep loss on breathing. *Journal of Applied Physiology* 1982;**53**:855–8.

9 Horne J A. The effects of sleep deprivation upon variations in heart rate and respiration rate. *Experientia* 1978;**33**:1175–6.

10 Naitoh P, Pasnau R O, Kollar E J. Psychophysiological changes after prolonged deprivation of sleep. *Biological Psychiatry* 1971;**3**:309–20.

11 Johnson L C, Slye E S, Dement W. Electroencephalographic and autonomic activity during and after prolonged sleep deprivation. *Psychosomatic Medicine* 1965;**27**:415–23.

12 Ross J J. Neurological findings after prolonged sleep deprivation. *Archives of Neurology* 1965;**12**:399–403.

13 Sassin J F. Neurological findings following short-term sleep deprivation. *Archives of Neurology* 1970;**22**:54–6.

14 Horne J A. Binocular convergence in man during total sleep deprivation. *Biological Psychology* 1975;**3**:309–19.

15 Wilkinson R T. Sleep deprivation. In: Edholm O G, Bacharach A L, eds. *Physiology of Survival*. London: Academic Press, 1965:399–430.

16 Naitoh P. Sleep deprivation. *Waking and Sleeping* 1976;**1**:53–60.

17 Ellingson R J, Wilken K, Bennett D R. Efficacy of sleep deprivation as an activation procedure in epilepsy patients. *Journal of Clinical Neurophysiology* 1984;**1**:83–101.

18 Vogel G W. Evidence for REM sleep deprivation as the mechanism of action of antidepressant drugs. *Progress in Neuropsychopharmacology and Biological Psychiatry* 1983;**7**:343–9.

19 Gillin J C. The sleep therapies of depression. *Progress in Neuropsychopharmacology and Biological Psychiatry* 1983;**7**:351–4.

20 Johnson L C. Sleep deprivation and performance. In: Webb W B, ed. *Biological Rhythms, Sleep and Performance*. New York: Wiley, 1982:111–42.

21 Morris G O, Williams H L, Lubin A. Misperception and disorientation during sleep deprivation. *Archives of General Psychiatry* 1960;**2**:247–54.

22 Horne J A. Human sleep and tissue restitution: some qualifications and doubts. *Clinical Science* 1983;**65**:569–78.

23 Horne J A, Wilkinson S. Chronic sleep reduction: daytime vigilance performance and EEG measures of sleepiness, with particular reference to practice effects. *Psychophysiology* 1985;**22**:69–78.

24 Adam K, Oswald I. Protein synthesis, body renewal and the sleep-wake cycle. *Clinical Science* 1983;**65**:561–7.

25 Waterlow J C, Garlick P J, Milward D J. *Protein Turnover in Mammalian Tissues and in the Whole Body*, Amsterdam: Elsvier, 1978.

26 Scheving L E. Mitotic activity in the human epidermis. *Anatomical Record* 1959;**135**:7–20.

27 Horne J A. The effects of exercise on sleep: a critical review *Biological Psychology* 1981;**7**:55–102.

28 Horne J A, Staff L H E. Exercise and sleep: body heating effects. *Sleep* 1983;**6**:36–46.

29 Horne J A, Moore V J. Sleep effects of exercise with and without additional body cooling. *Electroencephalography and Clinical Neurophysiology* 1985;**60**:33–8.

30 Shapiro C M, Goll C C, Cohen G R, Oswald I. Heat production during sleep. *Journal of Applied Physiology* 1984;**56**:671–7.

31 Wilkinson R T. Sleep deprivation: performance tests for partial and selective sleep deprivation. In: Abt L E, Reiss B F, eds. *Progress in Clinical Psychology: Vol 3 Dreams and dreaming*. London: Grune and Stratton, 1968:28–43.

32 Friedmann J K, Globus G G, Huntley A, Mullaney D J, Naitoh P, Johnson L C. Performance and mood during and after gradual sleep reduction. *Psychophysiology* 1977;**14**:245–50.

33 Benoit O, Foret J, Bouard G, Merle B, Landau J, Marc M E. Habitual sleep length and patterns of recovery sleep after 24 hour and 36 hour sleep deprivation. *Electroencephalography and Clinical Neurophysiology* 1980;**50**:477–85.

34 Gagnon P, De Koninck J, Broughton R. Reappearance of EEG slow waves in extended sleep with delayed bedtime. *Sleep* 1985;**8**:118–28.

35 Webb W B, Agnew H W. Are we chronically sleep deprived? *Bulletin of the Psychonomic Society* 1975;**6**:47–8.

36 Velasco F, Velasco M, Cepeda C, Munoz H. Wakefulness-sleep modulation of cortical and sub-cortical somatic evoked potentials in man. *Electroencephalography and Clinical Neurophysiology* 1980;**48**:64–72.

DISCUSSION

Audience   Dr Horne, do you have any views on sleep deprivation in the treatment of affective disorders?

Dr Horne   This is becoming very popular in the States although it is a controversial area. The tricyclic antidepressants suppress REM sleep and are also efficacious in treating certain forms of depression. The Americans thought that if they deprived people of REM sleep by waking them up when they have REM sleep this would improve the depression. There is evidence that this is the case. It now seems that it is not REM sleep deprivation which is the factor, but reducing sleep. The current state of the art, as espoused by Drs Gerald Vogel and Chris Gillin,[18,19] is that if sleep is shortened to 4 hours per night there is some benefit in severe forms of endogenous depression. There appears to be wide individual differences, but this shortened sleep regimen may be worth trying.

Dr Stradling   What is the suggested mechanism?

Dr Horne   It is attributed to various brain chemicals, but no one really knows which ones. It is certainly not related to REM sleep supression specifically. The idea that REM sleep suppression is the factor whereby the tricyclics are effective, is not now supported. Interestingly, some of the newer tricyclics do not suppress REM sleep, but are still efficacious in the treatment of depression.

Audience   Dr Horne, concerning your comments on recovery sleep after deprivation, the fact that lost slow wave sleep is almost entirely made up and REM only partially so, does that suggest that the 2 different types of sleep have different functions?

Dr Horne   One must be careful about saying one sleep has one function, another sleep has another; there must be interacting functions between these. My personal view is that in slow wave sleep, the delta waves represent some sort of cerebral recovery function essential for the brain, particularly for the frontal areas. On the other hand perhaps REM sleep stimulates the brain periodically throughout sleep to test the circuits, and in this respect, is possibly a substitute for wakefulness, following the repair processes of deep sleep. Maybe this is why you can replace much of REM sleep by wakefulness with little ill effect. REM sleep may not be a vital function for the brain. Tricyclics may reduce REM sleep to 5% in people who have depression, and there is no sign of neurological or cerebral defect as a result of lacking REM sleep, even over long periods of time.

Dr Adam, Vice Chairman of the Junior Hospital Doctors Association Is there any evidence that sleep deprivation in junior hospital doctors could cause them to make clinical mistakes?

Dr Horne In the study of sleep deprivation, many of the tests that have been used are simple and not very subtle, like reaction time. This can be performed just as well under limited sleep loss, if the subject simply tries harder. In my laboratory, we are now finding that by using subtle neuropsychological tests, particularly those that tap flexible or 'lateral' thinking ability, then one night's sleep loss has a significant effect here. People perseverate more—they revert to ineffective routines which they know are wrong, but despite their best efforts, they cannot get out of this 'rut' in their thinking. More tests need to be developed, especially those that assess verbal skills. Sleep loss certainly causes paucity in speech, and people have more difficulty in expressing what they mean. This is an area requiring much more investigation, and is very relevant to the work of junior hospital doctors.

LIST OF DELEGATES
SLEEP DISORDERS SYMPOSIUM
1st July 1988

Acharyya P
Newcastle under Lyme

Adams G P
London

Ah-Sien K L
Slough

Alani S M
Salford

Ananthanarayanan T S
Stoke on Trent

Angel J H
Watford

Archer G J
Stockport

Armstrong M A
Lincoln

Aylard C
Ilkeston

Bartlet L
Southampton

Bergel N
Oxford

Bhuiyan M A
Derby

Bird J
St Albans

Blackburn M
Horsham

Bruce M S
London

Christian M T A
Kettering

Coe J A
Ilkeston

Cohen R
Enfield

Conway C G
Ivybridge

Critchlow S G
London

Crutchfield M
London

Culliford L D
Sutton

Davys M
London

De A
Barrow in Furness

De-Pauw K W
Leicester

De Saram E M R
Chesterfield

Diaper P
Portsmouth

Disley D
Oxford

Dobbs R J
Harrow

Dobbs S M
Harrow

Dominian J
London

Dowling E
Norwich

Duncan A
Manchester

France R
Camberley

Franklin M
London

Gannon L E
Warwick

Ghosh S K
Hereford

Green G M
Norwich

Gregory C A
Oxford

Halford P
London

Holland R L
Dagenham

Holman C J
London

Hudman P
London

Husain A
Walsall

Hussain E S
Southport

Hussain Haye S
Karachi

Idzikowski C
Wantage

Ijaz Q
Fareham

Iqbal M
Birmingham

Jeganathan N
Nottingham

John A C
Carshalton

Joseph I
Caterham

Keet J
London

Kember M J
Enfield

Klijnsma M P
Canterbury

Leslie N D G
Hitchin

Lever N
Epsom

Lucas V
Cheam

Macdonald D W
Redruth

Mace C J
London

Mason I
Woking

McCarthy N
London

McKirdy A
Haywards Heath

Mell A
Wakefield

Merson S R
London

Miller P D
Borehamwood

Musch B
France

Nicol A
Bristol

Nicholson P W
Harrow

Noble I
Barnsley

Osman E E
Lincoln

Perera V T
Barnsley

Poon C M
Barnet

Prothero W B F
Ashford, Middlesex

Pusavat L T
London

Rabee S
London

Resek G
London

Reza H
Southampton

Robertson D N
Lincoln

Robin A A
Richmond

Roebuck M
Barnsley

Rose L
London

Salem S A M
Lincoln

Sedgewick P
London

Sharpley A
Oxford

Sharrard H E
Bristol

Solomon R
Oxford

Stanley S
Poole

Stores G
Oxford

Sudbury P R
London

Suleman N A
Bournemouth

Szulecka T K
Worksop

Tamby R
Bedford

Tangye S R
London

Taylor R
London

Welch C B
Ashford, Middlesex

Williams P
Oxford

Yang J D
Oxford

Zaiwalla Z
Oxford

Zaman M A
Derby

MEDICAL RELATIONS PUBLICATIONS

Current Approaches Series

Nutrition in the Elderly
Bulimia Nervosa
Aspects of Vertigo
Small Bowel Disease
Alzheimer's Disease
Renal Failure
Endometrial Carcinoma
ECT
Risk/Benefits of Antidepressants
Obesity
The Biological Clock
Affective Disorders in the Elderly

Occasional Papers/Supplements

Acquired Subglottic Stenosis in Infants
(Supplement No. 17 *Journal of Laryngology and Otology*—November 1988)

The above publications can be obtained by writing to:

Duphar Medical Relations
Duphar Laboratories Limited
West End
Southampton SO3 3JD